- HORMONAL HARMONY-
DEMYSTIFYING MEPOPAUSE HORMONE THERAPY

Hormone Therapy Isn't About Defying Age; It's About Empowering Women to Live Healthier, Balanced and Vibrant Lives Post-Menopause

DINESH KANFADE

ACKNOWLEDGEMENTS

I wish to express my gratitude to various sources, knowingly or unknowingly has contributed for empowering my knowledge, empowering women's health and helping me to write this book.

I would like to thank my mentors and teachers who had been a torch bearer for me for writing this book.

I am extremely thankful to **Dr. Parag Biniwale,** Sr. Consultant Obstetrics & Gynecology for taking time from his busy schedule to write **"FOREWORD"** for my book.

Book images Credit and Courtesy: *

Anatomical and Physiological Changes in GSM:

Source: Johnston L. The Recognition and Management of Atrophic Vaginitis. *Geriatrics and Aging 2002;5(7):9-15*

I also express my sincere gratitude to my family members and friends who have always been supportive and motivated me in my initiatives in writing series of books on **"Women's Health"**, this book being tenth in the series.

DEDICATION

Dedicated to my better half Nita,

son Akshay, daughter-in-law Priya

and little sweet Avni.

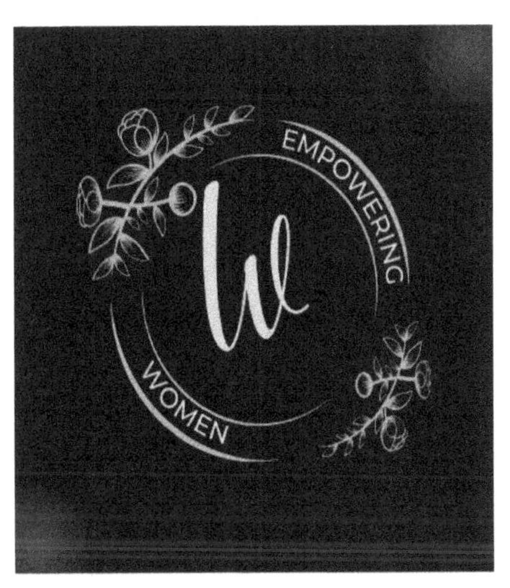
EMPOWERING
W
WOMEN

"A doctor's mission should not be to prevent death, but more importantly it should be to improve the quality of life."

- Abhijit Naskar

A happy woman is happy, not because everything is happy in her life. She is happy because her attitude towards everything in her life is right.

- Anonymous

FOREWORD

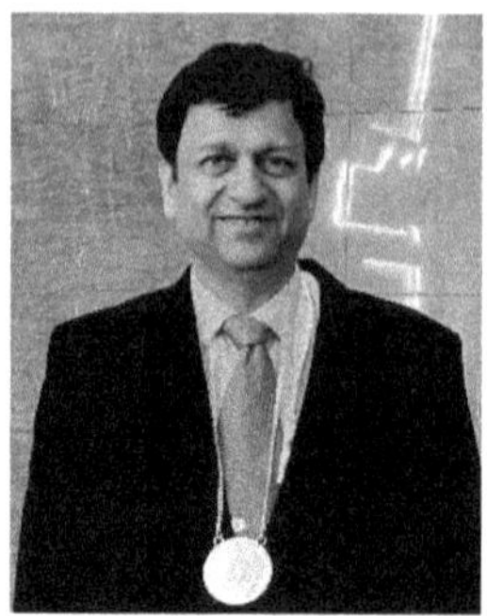

It is an honor to pen this foreword for such a well-crafted and thoughtful work.

Menopause is a natural transition in every woman's life and with increased longevity almost one third of a woman's life is spent in hormone-depleted phase. Menopause is a phase of life with complexities often leave many with unanswered questions and unnecessary anxiety. In the midst of widespread myths and misconceptions, hormone therapy emerges as one of the most debated solutions. It is in this context that ***"Demystifying Menopause Hormone Therapy"*** becomes an invaluable guide – a book that offers clarity and empowers women to make informed choices about their health and well-being.

Through well-structured chapters, the author provides practical insights into understanding hormonal changes, recognizing symptoms, and considering MHT as an option tailored to individual needs. With holistic approach, book also touches upon alternative therapies, lifestyle modifications, making it a comprehensive resource for healthcare professionals, caregivers, and women navigating this stage of life.

I would like to congratulate Dr. Dinesh Kanfade for coming out with a simplified version of Menopause Hormone Therapy. I am sure more and more clinicians would use it and make life much better for lot of women suffering from menopausal symptoms.

DR. PARAG BINIWALE

MD (Obst & Gyne), FICOG, FICMCH, Diploma in Pelviscopy (Germany)

Sr. Consultant, Ob / Gyn, Biniwale Women's Clinic, Pune

Unit Head & P G Teacher, Kamla Nehru Hospital

Chairman, Indian College of Obstetrics & Gynecology (ICOG) 2025

President, Menopause Society Pune (2018 – 22)

PREFACE

Menopause is a significant phase in every woman's life, bringing with it profound physiological and emotional changes. While this natural transition marks the end of reproductive years, it often introduces a range of challenging symptoms, including hot flashes, night sweats, mood swings and changes in bone density.

For decades, menopause hormone therapy has been a subject of both hope and controversy, leaving many women confused and apprehensive about its use.

The purpose of this book**, *"Demystifying Menopause Hormone Therapy",*** is to provide a comprehensive, evidence-based guide that helps women and healthcare professionals make informed decisions about managing menopausal symptoms effectively.

Throughout this book, I have strived to clarify the role of hormone therapy, addressing common myths, misconceptions, and safety concerns. The chapters are structured to offer a balanced perspective, beginning with an overview of menopause and its impact on health, followed by detailed discussions on different hormone therapy options, their benefits, risks and the latest advancements in the field. Practical tips on lifestyle modifications, alternative therapies, and selfcare strategies are also included to support holistic well-being during this stage.

With growing awareness about women's health and increasing life expectancy, understanding menopause and its management is more important than ever. Whether you are a woman approaching menopause, a healthcare provider, or a caregiver, this book ***"Demystifying Menopause Hormone Therapy"*** aims to serve as a valuable resource in navigating the complexities of hormone therapy with confidence.

DR. DINESH KANFADE

MBBS., DGO., DFP., FICMCH., CIMP.

Sr. Obstetrician & Gynecologist

TABLE OF CONTENT

CHAPTER I: INTRODUCTION

"No great progress has been made in

Science, Politics and Religion

without controversy"

-Anonymous

(A) Importance of Menopause Hormone Therapy

Menopausal Hormone Therapy (MHT) plays a pivotal role in managing menopausal symptoms and enhancing the quality of life for many women. Here's a systematic overview of its importance:

1. Alleviation of Vasomotor Symptoms

- **Hot Flashes and Night Sweats:** MHT is the most effective treatment for reducing the frequency and severity of hot flashes and night sweats, which are common during menopause.

2. Improvement of Urogenital Health

- **Vaginal Dryness and Atrophy:** MHT helps alleviate vaginal dryness, itching, and discomfort during intercourse by restoring the health of vaginal tissues.

- **Urinary Symptoms:** It can reduce the urinary urgency and frequency associated with menopausal changes after recurrent urinary tract infection is ruled out or treated with appropriate antibiotics.

3. Prevention of Osteoporosis

- **Bone Density Maintenance:** MHT helps prevent bone loss that occurs early in menopause when started before the age of 60 or within 10 years of menopause for severe hot flashes and night sweats, thereby reducing the risk of osteoporosis and fractures. ***(Bisphosphonates are recommended as first line therapy for osteoporosis).***

4. Cardiovascular Health

- **Heart Disease Risk Reduction:** When started before the age of 60 or within 10 years of menopause for severe hot flashes and night sweats, MHT may reduce the risk of heart disease. ***(MHT is not indicated for primary or secondary prevention of cardiovascular disease).***

5. Mood and Cognitive Function

- **Mood Stabilization:** MHT can help alleviate mood swings, depression, and irritability associated with menopause.

- **Cognitive Benefits:** Some studies suggest MHT may have a protective effect on cognitive function when initiated during the perimenopausal period for hot flashes and night sweats.

6. Skin and Hair Health

- **Skin Elasticity:** MHT can improve skin thickness and elasticity, reducing the appearance of wrinkles.

- **Hair Health:** It may help in reducing hair thinning and loss associated with hormonal changes.

7. Sexual Function

- **Libido Enhancement:** MHT can improve sexual desire and arousal, addressing sexual dysfunction that may occur during menopause.

- **Pain Reduction:** It alleviates pain during intercourse caused by vaginal dryness and atrophy.

8. Quality of Life

- **Overall Well-being:** By addressing multiple menopausal symptoms, MHT significantly enhances the overall quality of life for many women.

It's important to note that the benefits and risks of MHT vary among individuals. A thorough evaluation by a healthcare provider is essential to determine if MHT is appropriate for a specific individual.

(B) Historical Aspects of MHT

Understanding the historical development of MHT provides valuable context for its evolution, controversies, and current advancements. Here's a systematic breakdown:

1. Early Recognition of Menopause and Hormonal Deficiency

- **Ancient Times**
  - Menopause was recognized as a natural aging process but was poorly understood.
  - Treatments were largely based on herbal remedies and cultural practices.
- **19th Century**
  - Early medical literature described menopause as a "deficiency disease" requiring intervention.
  - Remedies included tonics, opium, and dietary changes.

2. Discovery of Hormones (Early 20th Century)

- **1900s: Identification of Estrogen**
  - Scientists began isolating and identifying ovarian hormones, notably estrogen.
  - Estrogen's role in regulating the menstrual cycle and alleviating menopause symptoms was discovered.

- **1920s–1930s: Hormonal Extraction**
    - Early forms of estrogen therapy involved crude extractions from animal sources, particularly adult female horse (mare) urine **(e.g., "Premarin").**
    - Limited understanding of long-term side effects which led to cautious use.

3. Rise of Hormone Therapy (Mid-20th Century)

- **1940s–1950s: Synthetic Estrogen**
    - Synthetic estrogens like diethylstilbestrol (DES) became available.
    - Estrogen was hailed as a **"youth hormone,"** rejuvenating women and alleviating menopausal symptoms.
- **1960s: Hormone Therapy Popularized**
    - **Dr. Robert A. Wilson's book, *Feminine Forever*,** promoted estrogen as a solution to menopause.
    - Estrogen therapy became widely marketed as a way to maintain youth, vitality, and femininity.

4. Emerging Concerns and Combined Hormone Therapy (1970s–1980s)

- **1970s: Cancer Concerns**
    - Studies linked estrogen-only therapy to an increased risk of endometrial cancer if started in woman with intact uterus.

    - This led to the development of combined hormone therapy (CHT), which included progestogens to counteract risks of endometrial cancer.

- **1980s: Expanded Use of Hormones**
    - MHT became a standard treatment for menopausal symptoms and prevention of osteoporosis.
    - Pharmaceutical companies heavily marketed hormone therapy as a long-term health solution.

5. The Women's Health Initiative (WHI) and its Impact (2000s)

- **2002: WHI Study Results**
    - The first clinical trial on hormone therapy (Conjugated Equine Estrogen 0.625 mg + Medroxyprogesterone acetate 2.5 mg / day) and to treat chronic menopausal conditions were started in USA between 1993 and 1998.
    - After the announcement of the first result of WHI 2000, MHT concerns involved three main issues: increased risk of breast cancer, increased risk of cardiovascular disease and increased risk of stroke with combined MHT.
    - The risk of both breast cancer and cardiovascular disease was significantly higher than the placebo risk. It left healthcare providers and consumers under the impression that all MHTs were bad in general.
    - Media created widespread panic over the safety of menopause hormone therapy and gave a clear message that MHT has more risks than benefits in

all women. Therefore, the MHT use was dramatically stopped.

- **The results, inferences and conclusions of WHI 2000 were based on the wrong approach to the use of MHT.**
  - ✓ **Approach to MHT was generalized.**
    - Age was not taken into consideration.
    - Fixed doses with fixed dose combinations to all patients.
    - Treatment continued for indefinite period.
    - No risk calculations before starting MHT.
  - ✓ **Prevention was given the upper hand over symptom relief.**
    - Long term treatment was given for prevention of chronic diseases e.g. coronary heart disease, osteoporosis, fractures, colon cancer.
    - Combination of Conjugated Equine Estrogen and Medroxyprogesterone acetate was used for MHT.
    - It was further realized that the increased risk of breast cancer was not due to estrogen, but the culprit was medroxyprogesterone acetate.

6. World Health Initiative 2013

- In the following years, reanalysis of WHI trials were performed and new studies showed that the use of MHT in perimenopausal and early menopausal women had beneficial effects.

- Subsequent publication of full WHI results, that supported MHT, were overlooked and were not highlighted by media.

- It took years to undo the damage done by badly interpreted publications in past.

- Almost a generation of women were mostly been denied the opportunity to improve quality of life post menopause.

7. World Health Initiative 2019:

- Final analysis, especially subgroup analysis and the subsequent publications of WHI shed a new light on the utility of MHT.

- The opinion and guidelines provided by the world's leading associations helped to place MHT in right perspective.

8. MHT today:

- Target population for initiation of therapy is within 10 years of menopause and below 60 years of age. MHT initiated early in symptomatic menopausal healthy women is always beneficial and safe.

- Emphasis on **"Timing Hypothesis"** suggests benefits always outweigh risks when therapy begins early in menopause.

- Prevention is out and symptomatic relief is in.

- Generalization is out while individualization is in. As one shoe is not suitable for all feet, similarly one fixed dose cannot be suitable for all women. Current approach is to individualize the therapy, the dose, the route, and the duration. Effective dose is started initially and titrated so as to relieve the symptoms.

- Micronized progesterone or Dydrogesterone preferred over Medroxyprogesterone acetate for prevention of endometrial hyperplasia in a combined regimen while starting MHT in a woman with intact uterus.

- Innovations like transdermal patches, gels and vaginal rings provided safer and more convenient options.

- Risk calculations are applied strictly:
    - Taking detailed history.
    - Physical examination, including breast and pelvis.
    - Basic mandatory investigations.
    - Special added investigations for some women, if indicated as per history.
    - Using "Risk Assessment Tools" for breast cancer and cardiovascular disease.
    - Using the right MHT, route, and duration of therapy. So finally:

"Right Woman, Right MHT, Right Dose,

and Right Duration

is the Right Approach for Prescribing MHT

so that Benefits far Outweigh the Risk."

9. Global Guidelines:

- International organizations (e.g., **North American Menopause Society, NICE, ACOG**) issued updated, nuanced guidelines.

- Indian Menopause Society (IMS) Guidelines: "Clinical Practice Guidelines on Menopause" in Indian context.

- **Menopause and MHT in 2024: addressing the key controversies – an International Menopause Society White Paper.** (https://doi.org/10.1080/13697137.2024.2394950)

- The International Menopause Society (established in 1970) in collaboration with the World Health Organization (WHO) has designated **October 18 as 'World Menopause Day' and month as 'Menopause Awareness Month.'** The global initiatives are dedicated to millions of mature women of 40 plus who are going to spend one-third of their life after menopause and are unaware or ignorant about the positive steps to be taken for improving their quality of life in the second inning.... **the postmenopausal life.**

- Indian Menopause Society (established in 1995) with its member societies are trying hard to sensitize the healthcare providers especially the practicing gynecologists towards the health of menopausal women in promoting the concept of menopausal clinics all over India.

This historical framework highlights the evolution of MHT, underscoring its scientific progress and challenges. It sets the stage for discussions on current practices, advancements, and the way forward in menopausal care.

(C) Misconceptions in Relation to MHT

To clarify common misunderstandings about MHT, this section systematically addresses key misconceptions and provides evidence-based facts to counter them.

Misconception 1: MHT Causes Breast Cancer in All Women

Fact:

- MHT, particularly combined hormone therapy (estrogen + progestogen), has been associated with a slight increase in breast cancer risk after 3–5 years of use.
- The risk of developing breast cancer is again minimized by using micronized progesterone or dydrogesterone instead of Medroxyprogesterone Acetate (MPA) in combined regimen.
- However, estrogen-only therapy (for women without a uterus) shows little to no increased risk of breast cancer and may even lower it in some cases.
- The risk varies based on factors such as age, timing of therapy, duration, and type of hormones used.
- Breast cancer risk from MHT is so low that it can be comparable to risks associated with lifestyle factors like obesity, sedentary lifestyle or alcohol consumption.

Misconception 2: MHT Is Unsafe for All Women

Fact:

- MHT is safe and beneficial for most healthy women under 60 or within 10 years of menopause onset.
- Risks increase with age and time since menopause, but the **"Timing Hypothesis"** supports its safety when started early.

- Modern formulations and delivery methods, such as transdermal patches and vaginal preparations, significantly reduce risks compared to older treatments.

Misconception 3: MHT Is Only for Severe Symptoms

Fact:

- While MHT is highly effective for managing severe symptoms like hot flashes and night sweats, it also provides other health benefits.
    - Prevents osteoporosis and reduces fracture risk.
    - Improves urogenital health, reducing vaginal dryness and urinary symptoms.
    - May have cognitive and cardiovascular protective effects when started early.
    - Women with moderate symptoms or those seeking long-term health benefits may also consider MHT.

Misconception 4: MHT Increases Heart Attack and Stroke Risk for Everyone

Fact:

- Combined results from studies like the Women's Health Initiative (WHI) initially suggested increased cardiovascular risks, leading to fear.
- Reanalysis of data shows that risks depend on timing:
    - **Early Use:** MHT started within 10 years of menopause may reduce the risk of heart disease.
    - **Late Use:** MHT initiated many years after menopause can increase cardiovascular risks.
- Transdermal estrogen (patches, gels) and lower-dose therapies are associated with a reduced risk of blood clots and strokes compared to oral formulations.

Misconception 5: MHT Causes Weight Gain

Fact:

- Weight gain during menopause is primarily due to aging and metabolic changes, not MHT.
- Studies indicate MHT may help redistribute body fat and prevent central obesity, common during menopause.
- Proper lifestyle adjustments in combination with MHT can counteract weight gain.

Misconception 6: Natural or Herbal Remedies Are Safer Than MHT

Fact:

- "Natural" doesn't always mean safer or more effective.
- Herbal and dietary supplements are often unregulated, with inconsistent quality and limited evidence of efficacy.
- Bioidentical hormones are sometimes marketed as "natural" but are subject to similar risks as standard MHT unless properly compounded and prescribed.

Misconception 7: MHT Should Be Taken Indefinitely

Fact:

- MHT is typically recommended for symptom relief and bone health during a specific time frame, often for 3–5 years or until the symptoms subside.
- Long-term use may be considered for some women with persistent symptoms or high risk of osteoporosis, under medical supervision.
- Regular evaluations are necessary to reassess the need for continuing therapy.

Misconception 8: MHT is Only for Women in Natural Menopause

Fact:

- MHT is also suitable for women experiencing early or surgical menopause (e.g., due to hysterectomy or oophorectomy).
- These women often benefit significantly from MHT as they face higher risks of osteoporosis, cardiovascular disease, and other health issues due to premature estrogen loss.

Misconception 9: MHT Increases the Risk of Dementia

Fact:

- Early concerns from studies like WHI suggested a potential link between MHT and dementia in older women.
- However, subsequent research shows that starting MHT during the perimenopause or early postmenopause years may have protective effects on cognitive function.
- Late initiation of MHT (after age 65) may be associated with a higher risk of dementia, emphasizing the importance of timing hypothesis.

Misconception 10: All Women Experience the Same Risks and Benefits

Fact:

- MHT effects are highly individualized, depending on factors like age, overall health, type of hormones, and delivery method.
- Personalized approaches to MHT help maximize benefits while minimizing risks.
- Consulting a healthcare provider ensures an informed and tailored decision.

Misconception 11: MHT Is Obsolete

Fact:

- Despite initial fears from the WHI study, MHT has undergone extensive re-evaluation, and its benefits are well-recognized today.
- Current guidelines support its use for symptom relief and health protection in appropriately selected women.
- Advances in formulations and delivery methods make MHT safer and more effective than ever.

By addressing these misconceptions with clear, evidence-based facts, healthcare providers and women will be empowered to make informed decisions about MHT and dispel undue fears.

(D) Objective and Target Audience of the Book

Objectives:

- **Educate Women About Menopause and MHT**
  - Provide comprehensive knowledge about menopause, its symptoms, and hormonal changes.
  - Explain how MHT can alleviate symptoms and improve quality of life.

- **Promote Evidence-Based Decision Making**
  - Clarify myths and misconceptions surrounding hormone therapy.
  - Present the latest research and clinical guidelines in an accessible manner.

- **Empower Women to Make Informed Choices**
  - Equip readers with knowledge about the risks, benefits, and alternatives to MHT.
  - Encourage shared decision-making between patients and healthcare providers.

- **Serve as a Resource for Healthcare Professionals**
  - Offer detailed clinical insights for gynecologists, general practitioners, and nurses.
  - Highlight the importance of personalized treatment plans and patient-centered care.

- **Bridge the Gap Between Research and Practice**
  - Simplify complex medical information for non-medical readers.
  - Showcase advancements in MHT, including bioidentical hormones and individualized approaches.

- **Promote Holistic Menopausal Care**
  - Address lifestyle, non-hormonal alternatives, and complementary therapies.

- Highlight emotional and mental health aspects of menopause.

- **Inspire Confidence in MHT**
  - Share real-life patient stories and testimonials to build trust and relatability.
  - Offer a roadmap for navigating menopause with or without MHT.

Target Audience of the Book: "Menopausal Hormone Therapy (MHT)"

- **Primary Audience: Women Experiencing Menopause**
  - Women in perimenopause, menopause, or postmenopause phases seeking symptom relief.
  - Individuals looking for clear, evidence-based guidance on MHT.

- **Healthcare Professionals**
  - Gynecologists seeking updated information on MHT.
  - General practitioners, family physicians, and nurse practitioners managing menopausal patients.

- **Medical Students and Residents**
  - Professionals preparing for clinical rotations or board exams.

- **Caregivers and Family Members**
  - Spouses, children, or caregivers who want to better understand menopause and support their loved ones.

- **Advocates of Women's Health**
  - Bloggers, influencers, or activists promoting women's health and wellness.

- Nonprofit organizations focused on menopause awareness and education.

CHAPTER II: UNDERSTANDING MENOPAUSE

"Menopause is a natural evolution,

a time to honor your journey and prepare

for new adventures."

– Anonymous

(A) Definition:

- Menopause is defined by Stedman as permanent cessation of menses. An awareness of menopause can be traced from ancient Greeks. In fact, the word menopause is derived from the Greek word meno meaning month and refers to menstrual cycle, while pause meaning to cease or to stop. In other words, menopause literally means cessation of monthly cycles.

- **The World Health Organization (WHO)** has defined natural menopause as the permanent cessation of menses resulting from loss of ovarian follicular activity. Menopause marks the end of reproductive life and natural menopause is the retrospective clinical diagnosis which occurs after 12 consecutive months of amenorrhoea, for which no other pathological cause can be established.

- The menopausal transition is the time before the final menopausal period **(FMP)** and is associated with irregular cycles, hormonal instability and symptoms.

(B) Pathophysiology of Menopause Transition:

- **Biology of ovarian aging:**

  In the human ovary, there is a continuous and progressive decline in the number of follicles from foetal life onwards. From several million follicles present at birth, less than a thousand remain at menopause. The loss cannot be accounted for by ovulation alone. Because the reproductive span of 30-35 years in a woman can only account for a loss of 350-450 ovarian follicles through ovulation. Their disappearance is also related to a loss of oocytes and surrounding granulosa and theca cells of the ovarian follicles that occur continuously through a process of follicular atresia. In every cycle, from a recruited pool of growing follicles, only one dominant follicle is selected, the rest undergoing atresia. It is clear from several studies **(Block 1952, Gougeon 1984, Gosden 1985, Richardson et al 1987)** that serum gonadotropins mainly follicular stimulating hormone (FSH) are responsible for accelerating the pace of follicular atresia leading to the depletion of stock and subsequent menopause.

- **Menopause Markers (Hormonal Changes during menopause transition):**

  The transition from the ovulatory cycles to the menopausal state is usually not an instantaneous event. Rather it is a series of hormonal clinical alterations that reflect declining ovarian function. Menopause is diagnosed retrospectively by history. Markers for diagnosis of menopause are preferably restricted for use in special situations and for fertility issues.

- **FSH** > 10 IU/L is indicative of declining ovarian function.

- **FSH** > 20 IU/L is diagnostic of ovarian failure in the perimenopausal age group with vasomotor symptoms (VMS) even in the absence of complete cessation of menses.

- **FSH** > 40 IU/L done 2 months apart is diagnostic of menopause.

- **FSH** rise precedes the LH rise.

- **FSH** is a diagnostic marker of ovarian failure while **LH** is not.

- **LH** measurement is not necessary to make a diagnosis of menopause.

- 1 - 3 years after menopause, serum **LH** rises by **3 folds** while **FSH** by **10 - 20 folds.** Rise in serum **LH** level is less pronounced than serum **FSH** level because **LH** has a shorter half-life period and has no specific negative peptide. **(FSH has a specific negative feedback peptide called Inhibin.)**

- **Postmenopausal serum estradiol level falls and it is < 20 pg/ml at menopause.** (Premenopausal level of serum estradiol varies from 40 -400 pg/ml).

- **AMH** and **Inhibin** levels are low or undetectable at menopause. Inhibin is a polypeptide that is secreted by granulosa cells, it has both paracrine and endocrine functions. At the central level inhibin exerts a negative feedback effect and reduces the pituitary secretion of FSH. At the ovarian level its paracrine function is to prevent folliculogenesis of other follicles. An increasing level of serum FSH during early follicular phase and a decline in circulating levels of inhibin and estradiol are the first indications of age-related acceleration of follicular depletion. Serum inhibin during the early follicular phase showed a significant decline in women of 45-49 years of age as compared to those aged below 45 years **(McLachlan et.al. 1987-88).**

- On transvaginal ultrasound the antral follicular count is low and ovarian volume is also reduced.

- **Estrogen/Testosterone Shift in Menopausal Women and other related factors:**

  During menopause, significant hormonal changes occur in women's body, particularly involving estrogen and testosterone. This Estrogen/Testosterone shift has profound effect on both physical and mental health.

  - **Estrogen Decline:** Normal serum estradiol level in women in reproductive age group is 40 – 400 pg/ml depending up on the stage of menstrual cycle. Estrogen is a key hormone in female sexual health. It is responsible for maintaining the health of vaginal tissues, promoting lubrication and supporting the overall sexual response cycle. Estradiol level in postmenopausal women is below 20 pg/ml. After menopause, ovaries no longer produce estrogen. Instead, in small amounts it is produced in a number of extra-gonadal sites such as kidney, adipose tissue, skin and brain. Unlike ovarian synthesized estrogen, which is released into the blood stream, estrogen synthesized within these extra-gonadal sites mostly acts locally at the site of synthesis and functions as a paracrine and/or intracrine factor to maintain important tissue specific functions.

- **Impact on Body:**
  - ✓ **Vasomotor Symptoms:** The decline in estrogen is responsible for common menopausal symptoms such as hot flashes and night sweats.

  - ✓ **Bone Health:** Reduced estrogen levels lead to decreased bone density, increasing the risk of osteoporosis.

  - ✓ **Cardiovascular Health:** Estrogen has protective effects on the heart and blood vessels; its decline can lead to an increased risk of cardiovascular diseases.

  - ✓ **Mental Health:** Estrogen influence neurotransmitter systems that regulate mood and cognitive functions. Its decrease can lead to symptoms such as depression, anxiety and cognitive decline.

- **Relative Increase in Testosterone:** While testosterone levels also decline during menopause, the decrease is more gradual compared to estrogen. As a result, there is a relative increase in androgen-to-estrogen ratio. This shift can lead to noticeable changes in a woman's body.

- **Effect of the Estrogen / Testosterone Shift:**
  - ✓ **Androgenic Symptoms:** The relative increase in testosterone can cause symptoms such as thinning scalp hair, increased facial hairs and a deeper voice.

- ✓ **Libido Changes:** Testosterone plays a role in sexual desire, and the hormonal shift during menopause can lead to changes in libido, with some women experiencing a decrease and others in increase in sexual interest.
- ✓ **Muscle Mass:** Testosterone helps maintain muscle mass, so while overall muscle mass may decline with aging, the relative increase in testosterone can help in preserving it to some extent.

- **Overall Impact:**
  The estrogen/testosterone shift during menopause contribute to a range of physical and mental health changes. The decline in estrogen is primarily responsible for the more commonly recognised symptoms of menopause, such as hot flashes, mood swings and increased risk of **osteoporosis** and cardiovascular issues. Meanwhile, because of relative increase in testosterone, there is emergence of androgenic symptoms.

- **Changes in cycle length and menstrual bleeding**:
  Women aged 18-24 years have an average follicular phase length of 15 ± 2 days, but those aged 40 -44 years have an average length of 10 + 2 days, which tends to shorten the menstrual cycle. Thus, menstrual cycle length may shorten before it lengthens as women progress through the transition. **(Trealar et. al. 1967).**

- One hallmark of the menopause transition is a change in bleeding pattern, **Van Voorhis and et. al**. has studied hormonal pattern and menstrual bleeding pattern in a large sub cohort of the **SWAN** participants aged 42-52 years. They found that 20% of all cycles during the time were anovulatory. They also noted that short cycle lengths (<21 days) were common early in menopause transition whereas long cycle intervals (> 36 days) were associated with late menopause transition.

(C) Age at Menopause:

- The menopause transition most often begins between ages 45 and 55 years. The average age at menopause of an Indian woman is 46.2 years, much less than western woman (51 years).
- From available Indian data it is hypothesized that an early age at menopause in Indian women (46.2 years) predisposes them to chronic health disorders a decade earlier than the Caucasians having late age at menopause (51 years).
- It is reported that osteoporotic fractures occur 10-20 years earlier in Indians as compared to Caucasians.
- The first myocardial infarction (MI) attack occurs in 4.4% of Asian women at a younger age than in European women.
- In India, type II diabetes occurs a decade earlier than the Caucasians.
- Breast cancer is the most common cancer in Indian women and the incidence peaks before the age of 50 years.

As the women approach their mid-forties, many women find themselves looking for signs of menopause and trying to figure out when it will begin for them. Most women reach menopause between the ages of 45 and 55 years. But as every woman is unique, age at menopause may also differ due to underlying conditions.

- **Genetic factors:**
  Research has conclusively shown that there is a strong link between menopause and genetics. There are approximately 50% chances that a woman will become menopausal at the same age as her mother or within a few years of that age. However, this may not always be the case.

- **Ethnicity:**
  Studies have conclusively revealed that the average menopausal age for Caucasian women in the UK and USA is around 51 years, while in Indians it is 46.2 yrs. The reason for these variations is that women of different ethnicities often have different levels of estrogenic activity.

- **Smoking**:
  Smoking has been found to be the number one modifiable lifestyle factor relating to early menopause. Polycyclic aromatic hydrocarbons found in cigarette smoke are toxic to ovarian follicles. These chemicals can cause premature loss of follicles leading to early onset of menopause.
  Smoking can lead to faster breakdown of oestrogen in the liver which in turn results in an earlier decline in oestrogen level.

- **Body Mass Index (BMI)**:
  A study conducted by Australian University has shown that women who are underweight or have a low BMI are more likely to enter menopause early, while women who are overweight or have high BMI are more likely to experience a late menopause. This is due to the fact that oestrogen is stored in fat cells.

- **Parity**:
  Nulliparous women may experience an earlier

menopause while multiparty or a late first pregnancy may result in a later onset.

- **Other factors include:**
  Women with bilateral oophorectomy, exposure to radiotherapy or chemotherapy in premenopausal age experience early induced menopause.

- **Use of oral contraceptives** may delay the onset.

Is there a menopause age calculator?

All factors discussed above could help women to determine the appropriate age at menopause but there is no definite test to predict it. In a nutshell AMH levels indicate the number of follicles present in the ovaries and unlike FSH levels, AMH levels do not fluctuate with phases in menstrual cycles, which means that they can be used to determine the extent of ovarian reserve and thereby the approximate age at which menopause will occur.

(D) Terminologies in Relation to Menopause:

- **Natural Menopause:**
  It is recognised to have occurred after 12 months of amenorrhoea for which there are no obvious pathological causes.

- **Premenopause:**
  It is often used to refer to the entire reproductive period up to the final menstrual period (FMP).

- **Perimenopause**:
  It is the period immediately before 2 - 3 years and 1 year after FMP. It may last up to 3 - 5 yrs. The characteristics are:
  . Increasing serum FSH levels
  . Significantly reduced fertility
  . Erratic menstrual periods
  . Onset of menstrual symptoms
  (The term is used interchangeably with menopause transition.)

- **Climacteric:**
  It is interchangeably used with perimenopause and menopause transition. When associated with symptoms, it is called climacteric syndrome.

- **Postmenopause:**
  It is the span of life dating from the final menstrual period onwards regardless of whether the menopause was spontaneous or iatrogenic.

- **Premature Ovarian Insufficiency (POI):**
  Premature ovarian Insufficiency has replaced the term premature menopause. POI is described as amenorrhoea due to loss of ovarian function before the age of 40

years. It is a state of female hypergonadotrophic hypogonadism. Its incidence is 1%. It can manifest as primary amenorrhoea with onset before menarche or secondary amenorrhoea with onset after the establishment of natural menses. Criteria for diagnosis of POI as per ***European Society of Human Reproduction and Embryology (ESHRE 2015) is 'Elevated FSH levels > 25 IU/L on two occasions > 4 weeks apart'.***

- **Early Menopause**:
  It is the time span between the spontaneous or iatrogenic menopause occurring between 40 years of age and the accepted typical age of menopause for a given population (between 40 and 46.2 years in Indian population). Incidence is 5%.

- **Delayed Menopause:**
  It is not well defined but may be important in terms of increased problems associated with hyperestrogenism. It is two SDs above from the natural average age of menopause in a given population. In India, we may consider it to be 54 years or more.

- **Postmenopausal Bleeding (PMB):**
  It is the bleeding which occurs 12 months after the last menstrual period. However, it is recommended that any vaginal bleeding that occurs 6 months after the last menstrual period should be investigated.

- **Induced Menopause/Surgical Menopause**:
  It is the cessation of menses due to bilateral oophorectomy or iatrogenic ablation of ovarian function or hysterectomy.

(E) Staging of Menopause:

- The purpose of the staging system of this physiological event is to improve comparability of strategies and to facilitate clinical decision-making.
- In 1997, Anklesaria in India published a simple clinical method of staging of menopause to understand and to deal with the problems of transition phase and beyond.

Modified Anklesaria's IMS Consensus Group Staging

Menopause			
Stage I	Stage II A	Stage II B	Stage III
Roughly 2 years before menopause Early (Premenopausal symptoms): IA Vasomotor instability IB Early psychosomatic symptoms Menstrual problems	1 year after last period Atrophic changes Genitourinary Vasomotor Weight gain Osteopenia	Up to 5 years after menopause Intermediate (postmenopausal symptoms): Late psychosomatic and genital symptoms Sexual disorders Residual changes from stage II A osteopenia or osteoporosis	From 5 years postmenopausal till Late (postmenopausal) complications: Residual changes from stage II Ischemic heart changes Other late complications, e.g. Alzheimer's disease, Osteoporosis
PREVENT	TREAT	TREAT	PALLIATE

Window of Opportunity

Stages of Reproductive Ageing Workshop (STRAW):

- Founded in Seoul in 2001
- Gold standard for characterizing reproductive aging through menopause.
- STRAW (2001) aimed to classify women's life in 3 phases: Reproductive, Menopause Transition and Postmenopause.
- It proposed nomenclature and a staging system for ovarian aging including menstrual and qualitative hormonal criteria to define each stage.
- This was applicable only to healthy women.

STRAW 2001:

The Anchor stage is the Final Menstrual Period (FMP), 5 stages precede and 2 stages follow FMP.

Seven stages of normal reproductive aging in women

The STRAW staging system[†] — Final Menstrual Period (FMP)

Stages	-5	-4	-3	-2	-1	0	+1	+2
Terminology	Reproductive			Menopausal Transition			Postmenopause	
	Early	Peak	Late	Early	Late*		Early*	Late
				Perimenopause				
Duration of stage	Variable			Variable		(a) 1 yr	(b) 4 yrs	Until demise
Menstrual cycles	Variable to regular	Regular		Variable cycle length (>7 days) different from normal	≥2 skipped cycles and an interval of amenorrhea (≥60 days)	Amen x 12 mos	None	
Endocrine	Normal FSH		Elevated FSH	Elevated FSH			Elevated FSH	

*Stages most likely to be characterized by vasomotor symptoms. [†]Stages of Reproductive Aging Workshop, held in Park City, Utah, USA, July 23-24, 2001, sponsored by the American Society for Reproductive Medicine, the National Institute on Aging, the National Institute of Child Health and Human Development, and the North American Menopause Society.

Soules MR, et al. Fertil Steril. 2001 Nov; 76(5):874-8.

ASMPH Approach to a patient with menopausal symptoms 10

Research conducted during 10 years added advanced knowledge of the critical changes in hypothalamic pituitary ovarian function that occur before and after the final menstrual period (FMP).

STRAW-10:

Founded in Washington DC in 2011, 10 stages (3 new added).

The 2011 Stages of Reproductive Aging Workshop + 10 staging system for reproductive aging in women

	Menarche						FMP (0)			
Stage	-5	-4	-3b	-3a	-2	-1	+1a	+1b	+1c	+2
Terminology	REPRODUCTIVE				MENOPAUSAL TRANSITION			POSTMENOPAUSE		
	Early	Peak	Late		Early	Late	Early			Late
					Perimenopause					
Duration	*Variable*				*Variable*	1–3 years	2 years (1+1)		3-6 years	*Remaining lifespan*
PRINCIPAL CRITERIA										
Menstrual cycle	Variable to regular	Regular	Regular	Subtle changes in flow/ length	*Variable length* Persistent ≥7-day difference in consecutive cycles	Interval of amenorrhea of ≥60 days				
SUPPORTIVE CRITERIA										
Endocrine										
FSH			Low	Variable*	↑ Variable*	↑ >25 IU/L**	↑ Variable		Stabilizes	
AMH			Low	Low	Low	Low	Low		Very low	
Inhibin B				Low	Low	Low	Low		Very low	
Antral follicle count			Low	Low	Low	Low	Very low		Very low	
DESCRIPTIVE CHARACTERISTICS										
Symptoms						Vasomotor symptoms *Likely*	Vasomotor symptoms *Most likely*			*Increasing* symptoms of urogenital atrophy

*Blood draw on cycle days 2–5 ↑ = elevated

**Approximate expected level based on assays using current international pituitary standard

Reproduced with permission from Harlow et al. Copyright Elsevier Science Inc.

STRAW-10 Advantages:

- Regardless of age
- Demographic
- BMI or lifestyle characteristics

Not used in:

- Premature Ovarian Failure (POF)
- Hysterectomy
- Endometrial Ablation
- PCOS
- HIV-AIDS

- Tamoxifen therapy
- Cancer patients undergoing chemotherapy

Need for further Research:

- Improved characterization of the pattern, timing and level of reproductive biomarkers across nations is necessary, especially to provide data on the experience of women from low-resource countries.

- Research is needed to better understand the process of reproductive aging and appropriate staging criteria for women with PCOS and POI and those who have removed a single ovary and/or hysterectomy.

- Research is needed to better evaluate staging in women with chronic illness such as HIV infection and those undergoing cancer treatment.

(F) Symptoms of Menopause:

- About 20% of women have no symptoms at all, while 60% have mild to moderate symptoms. The remaining 20% have severe symptoms that interfere with their daily life.

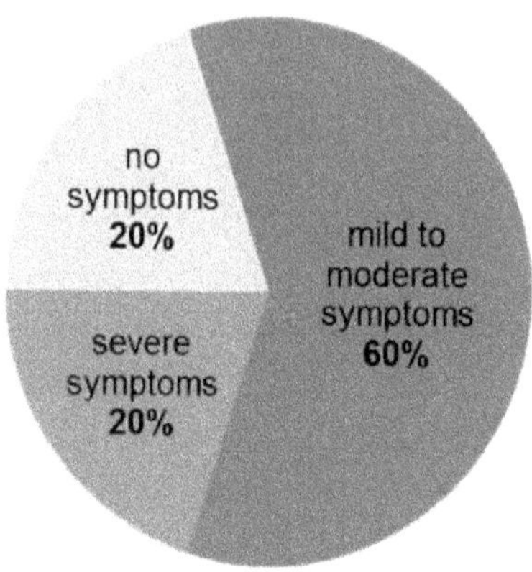

- Menopausal symptoms can be influenced by different factors, for example, your stage of life and general health and wellbeing.

- The biology and symptomatology of menopause is blurred due to its relationship to the underlying aging process.

- Vasomotor, urogenital symptoms and irregular menstrual periods are typically linked with serum oestrogen levels.

- Long term effects on bone and heart have been related to estrogen deficiency.

- Many other symptoms like muscle and joint pain, vertigo, mood changes, depression, insomnia, nervousness have been associated with menopause but are not necessarily due to decrease in oestrogen levels.

- Many symptoms start during perimenopause and can continue into postmenopause. Australian studies show that some women experience symptoms like hot flashes and night sweats well into their 60s.

Physical Symptoms:

Physical symptoms may include:

- Irregular periods
- Hot flashes
- Night sweats
- Sleep problems
- Sore breasts
- Itchy, crawly or dry skin
- Exhaustion and fatigue
- Dry vagina
- Loss of sex drive (libido)
- Headaches or migraine
- Aches and pains
- Bloating
- Urinary problems
- Weight gains due to androgen-estrogen ratio shift and low BMR.

Emotional symptoms may include:

- Feeling irritable or frustrated
- Feeling anxious
- Difficulty in concentrating
- Forgetfulness
- Mood swings

Symptoms and Disorders in Relation to Age and Menopause:

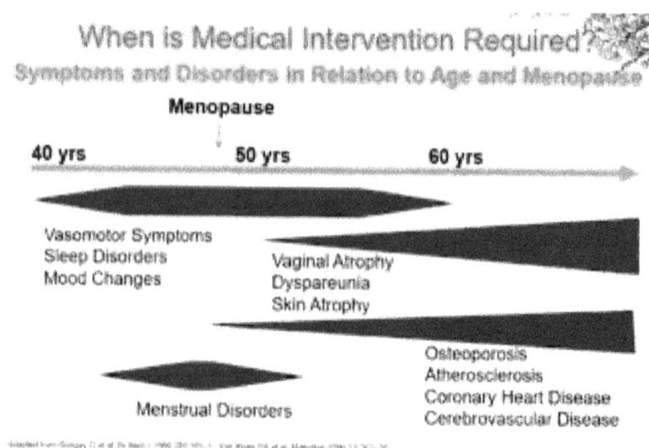

Source: Bungay G, et al. Br Med J 1980; 281: 181 - 3;

Van Keep PA, et al. Maturities 1990; 12:163-70.

- ***The immediate symptoms of menopause transition are irregular periods, hot flashes, night sweats, sleep and mood disturbances, joint and muscle pain, vaginal dryness and low sexual desire which generally resolve over a while in mild cases.***

- ***Genitourinary symptoms appear in the early postmenopausal period and may worsen over some time if not treated.***

- ***The long-term consequences of menopause affect bone and cardiovascular health which worsen with aging.***

CHAPTER III: WORK-UP FOR ASSESSING THE RISK FACTORS AT MENOPAUSE CLINIC

"Health is not just the absence of illness,

but the presence of well-being."

– Anonymous

(A) Importance of Menopause clinic:

With the global population aging rapidly, the establishment and accessibility of **menopause clinics** have become increasingly important. These clinics offer specialized care for women transitioning through menopause, addressing a variety of health concerns associated with this stage of life. Here are the key points highlighting their importance:

1. Growing Aging Population

- By 2050, the number of women aged 50 and older is projected to significantly increase, with many experiencing menopause and postmenopausal issues.
- Menopause clinics provide focused care, meeting the unique health needs of this demographic.

2. Management of Menopausal Symptoms

- Symptoms like **hot flashes, sleep disturbances, mood changes, and joint pain** can severely impact the quality of life.

- Menopause clinics offer evidence-based interventions, such as:
    - **Hormone replacement therapy (HRT)**
    - Non-hormonal therapies
    - Lifestyle modifications

3. Prevention of Chronic Diseases

Postmenopausal women face a higher risk of:

- **Osteoporosis**: Decline in estrogen levels increases bone density loss.
- **Cardiovascular diseases**: Menopause accelerates heart disease risk due to hormonal changes.
- **Diabetes and metabolic syndrome**: Menopause clinics focus on early identification and prevention of these conditions.
- **Prevention / Early Detection of Cancers:** Mainly cervical, endometrial, ovarian and breast cancers.

4. Mental and Emotional Support

- Emotional challenges like **anxiety, depression, and cognitive decline** are common during menopause.
- Clinics provide counseling, psychological support, and cognitive therapies to help women cope.

5. Enhancing Awareness and Education

- Menopause clinics serve as platforms to educate women about:
    - Symptoms and treatment options

- Lifestyle adjustments for healthy aging
- Importance of regular screenings (e.g., mammograms, bone density tests).

6. Personalized Care

- Every woman's experience of menopause is unique.
- Menopause clinics offer tailored treatment plans, including complementary and alternative therapies where appropriate.

7. Improved Quality of Life

- By addressing physical, emotional, and sexual health issues, menopause clinics empower women to maintain a high quality of life during and after menopause.

8. Contribution to Public Health

- As part of healthcare systems, menopause clinics reduce the burden of untreated symptoms, delayed diagnoses, and chronic diseases, contributing to healthier aging populations globally.
- The concept of menopausal health is about women getting and staying healthy throughout life and should celebrate postmenopausal life with strength, energy and certain goals.

The Centre for Disease Control and Prevention urges all women to make healthy living a priority.

In summary, the role of menopause clinics is pivotal in a world where the aging population is growing. They offer a **comprehensive, multidisciplinary approach** to address the health challenges faced by menopausal and postmenopausal women, ensuring that this significant demographic lives longer, healthier, and more fulfilling lives.

At menopause clinic primary healthcare provider is a gynecologist who takes detailed history, does physical examination including pelvic and breast examination, investigates her, identifies risk factors and formulate a plan for individualized counseling and treatment. The approach is basically multi-speciality oriented.

Here we will only discuss the points which are in relation with assessing the potential risk factors in relation to menopause, future risks of non-communicable diseases and health in general.

(B) History Taking:

1. Personal and Demographic Information

- Age: Chronological and menopausal age.
- Menopause Type: Natural, surgical, or premature menopause.
- Ethnicity: Relevant for assessing specific genetic or cultural risk factors.
- Occupation and Lifestyle: Sedentary or physically active, job stress.

2. Menstrual History

- Age at menarche.
- Age at menopause.
- Menstrual irregularities leading up to menopause.
- History of abnormal uterine bleeding.

3. Obstetric and Reproductive History

- Number of pregnancies, live births, miscarriages, or abortions.
- History of infertility or reproductive complications.
- Breastfeeding history.
- Use of hormonal contraception or fertility treatments.

4. Family History

- Cardiovascular diseases (e.g., hypertension, stroke).
- Osteoporosis or fractures.
- Breast, ovarian, or endometrial cancer.
- Diabetes mellitus or metabolic syndrome.
- Autoimmune disorders.

5. Medical History

- **Chronic Conditions:**
  - Cardiovascular disease.
  - Diabetes or prediabetes.
  - Osteoporosis or history of fractures.
  - Hypertension.
  - Thyroid disorders.
- **History of Cancer:**
  - Breast, ovarian, endometrial, or colon cancer.
- **Psychiatric History:**
  - Depression, anxiety, or mood disorders.
- **Other Conditions:**
  - Chronic kidney disease, liver disease, or autoimmune disorders.

6. Surgical History

- Hysterectomy (with or without oophorectomy).
- Surgeries for cancers or other gynecological conditions.
- Fracture repairs or joint replacements.

7. Lifestyle Factors

- Dietary Habits:
  - Calcium and vitamin D intake.
  - Diet quality and alcohol consumption.
- Physical Activity:
  - Sedentary vs active lifestyle.
- Smoking History:
  - Past or current smoking, duration, and intensity.
- Alcohol and Substance Use:
  - Type, frequency, and amount.

8. Gynecological and Breast History

- History of breast pain, lumps, or surgery.

- Use of hormone replacement therapy (HRT).
- History of sexually transmitted infections (STIs).
- Last Pap smear and mammogram.

9. Bone Health and Fracture Risk

- History of fractures or falls.
- Chronic joint or back pain.
- Use of glucocorticoids or other bone-impacting medications.

10. Cardiovascular Risk Assessment

- History of hypertension, dyslipidemia, or ischemic heart disease.
- Symptoms of angina or claudication.
- Obesity or central adiposity (waist circumference).

11. Metabolic Risk Factors

- History of metabolic syndrome, insulin resistance, or gestational diabetes.
- Weight changes during or after menopause.
- Symptoms of polycystic ovarian syndrome (PCOS).

12. Symptoms Related to Menopause

- Vasomotor symptoms: Hot flashes, night sweats.
- Genitourinary syndrome of menopause (GSM): Vaginal dryness, dyspareunia, or urinary issues.
- Sleep disturbances.
- Cognitive or memory concerns.
- Skin and hair changes.

13. Psychosocial and Sexual History

- Marital or relationship status.
- Sexual activity and satisfaction.

- Psychological well-being.
- Stress, coping mechanisms, or support systems.

14. Medication and Supplement History

- Current and past medications:
    - HRT or alternative therapies.
    - Calcium, vitamin D, or osteoporosis medications.
- Over-the-counter supplements.
- Complementary and alternative medicines.

15. Special Considerations

- Allergies or adverse reactions.
- Vaccination status (e.g., pneumococcal, influenza, shingles).
- Current or past infections impacting overall health.

This structured history-taking ensures comprehensive risk factor identification, aiding in personalized management and preventive strategies.

(C) Physical Examination:

A systematic **physical examination** at a menopause clinic is essential to evaluate overall health, identify risk factors, and detect existing diseases. Here's a detailed approach:

1. General Examination

Vital Signs:

- **Blood pressure:** Detect hypertension. (Normal B.P. 120/80 mm of Hg).

- **Heart rate and rhythm:** Identify arrhythmias or tachycardia. (A resting regular heart rate between 60 – 100 beats per minute is considered normal for most adults).

- **Respiratory rate:** Detect respiratory distress or abnormalities. (A normal respiratory rate for an adult at rest is 12 – 20 breaths per minute).

Body Weight and Height:

- **Body Mass Index (BMI):** Assess for obesity or underweight. (A healthy BMI range for women is 18.5 to 24.9, 25 to 29.9 overweight, 30 to 39.9 obese, 40 and above severe obese).

- **Waist-to-hip ratio:** Evaluate for central obesity - risk for metabolic syndrome and cardiovascular disease. (According to WHO, the average healthy waist-to-hip ratio for women is considered to be 0.8 or less).

2. Skin and Hair Examination

- **Skin**:
    - Look for dryness, thinning, or loss of elasticity (common in menopause).

- Inspect for pigmentation changes, bruising, or signs of systemic disease.

- **Hair**:
    - Check for alopecia or hirsutism.
    - Assess for hair thinning, which may indicate hormonal imbalance or nutritional deficiency.

3. Head and Neck Examination

- **Thyroid**:
    - Palpate for thyroid enlargement, nodules, or tenderness.
    - Assess for signs of hypothyroidism or hyperthyroidism.

- **Oral Cavity**:
    - Inspect for dental health, gum disease, and oral mucosa changes.
    - Look for signs of nutritional deficiencies (e.g., angular cheilitis, glossitis).

- **Eyes**:
    - Check for dryness or signs of vitamin A deficiency.
    - Assess for yellowing of sclera (liver disease).

- **Neck**:
    - Palpate lymph nodes for enlargement or tenderness.

4. Breast Examination

- **Inspection**:

- Observe for asymmetry, skin dimpling, or nipple discharge.
- Look for visible masses or skin changes.

- **Palpation**:
  - Perform systematic palpation to detect lumps, tenderness, or abnormalities.

- **Axillae**:
  - Palpate for lymphadenopathy.

5. Cardiovascular System Examination

- **Heart**:
  - Auscultate for murmurs, irregular rhythm, or other abnormalities.

- **Peripheral Circulation**:
  - Check for pulses in the extremities (e.g., dorsalis pedis, posterior tibial).
  - Assess for edema, varicose veins, or signs of vascular disease.

6. Respiratory System Examination

- Inspect chest wall movement and symmetry.

- Auscultate for breath sounds to detect wheezing, crackles, or reduced air entry.

- Look for signs of respiratory infections or chronic lung disease.

7. Abdominal Examination

- Inspect for abdominal distension, scars, or striae.

- Palpate for tenderness, masses, or organomegaly.

- Evaluate for hepatomegaly (liver disease) or splenomegaly.
- Check for signs of ascites.

8. Musculoskeletal and Bone Health

- Should include recording of height and weight annually. Also balance and gate to be checked.
- Get-up and Go test – by asking women to get-up from a chair without using their arms.
- Occiput to wall distance in standing position is ideally zero. Inability to touch occiput to the wall while standing indicates thoracic fracture.
- Inability to insinuate four fingers of the hand between the lower rib cage and anterior superior iliac crest indicates a lumbar fracture.
- Women presenting with fracture complain of severe pain, which is sudden in onset with minimal trauma.
- In Vitamin D deficiency, proximal muscles are affected more than the distal. So, activities such as using a squatting toilet, climbing stairs and getting out of a lower heighted chair can be particularly difficult.
- Tenderness on the tibia and sternum can be elicited.
- Kyphosis and Dowager's hump are seen at late stages of osteoporosis.

9. Genitourinary Examination

- **External Genitalia**:
  - Inspect for atrophy, lesions, or prolapse.

- **Vaginal Examination**:
  - Assess for vaginal atrophy, dryness, or infections.
  - Look for signs of pelvic organ prolapse.

- **Speculum Examination**:
  - Look for any abnormality in cervix.

- **Bimanual Palpation**:
  - Palpate for uterine or adnexal masses or tenderness.

- **Urinary Examination**:
  - Evaluate for stress incontinence, pelvic floor weakness, or bladder tenderness.

10. Neurological Examination

- Test reflexes, especially in the lower limbs (e.g., Achilles reflex).
- Assess balance and coordination (risk of falls or neurological disease).
- Evaluate for neuropathy symptoms (e.g., in diabetes or vitamin B12 deficiency).

11. Psychosocial and Cognitive Assessment

- Evaluate for signs of depression or anxiety (postmenopausal women are at risk).
- Assess cognitive function if concerns of memory loss or brain fog are reported.
- Look for signs of sleep disturbance or fatigue.

This comprehensive examination ensures early detection of risks and guides appropriate management strategies.

(D) Laboratory Tests:

Routine investigations include:

- **CBC**
  To detect anaemia, infection and other haematological disorders.
- **ESR / CRP**
  To assess for inflammation or chronic diseases.
- **VDRL**
- **HBsAg**
- **HIV**
- **Blood sugar F, Hb1Ac**
  Normal values Blood Sugar F: < 100 mg/dl
  HbA1C: Monitors long-term glucose control: Normal values: Between 4 – 5.6 %. Levels between 5.7 and 6.4 suggest that you are prediabetes and a higher chance of getting diabetes.
- **Lipid profile**
  Normal values:
    - Total Cholesterol: < 200 mg/dl
    - Triglycerides: < 150 mg/dl
    - LDL-C: < 100 mg/dl
    - HDL-C: > 40 mg/dl
- Liver Function Tests (LFT)
- Renal Function Tests (RFT)
- Thyroid Function Tests (T3, T4, TSH)
- Serum Calcium
  Normal values: Between 8.5 – 10.5 mg/dl
- 25 OH Vit D
  Normal values: 30 – 60 ng/mL
- Parathyroid Hormone (PTH), if necessary.

Following investigations are not mandatory and should be advised judiciously depending up on history and physical examination:

- Hormonal studies
- Coagulation studies
- Endometrial sampling
- Measurement of bone mineral density by DEXA
- Urodynamic studies

(E) Screening for Common Cancers in Women

1. Cervical Cancer:

Cervical cancer screening is a critical component of preventive healthcare services offered at menopause clinics. Given that many women at menopause are at an age where routine screening is essential, menopause clinics serve as a valuable point of care to identify and manage cervical cancer risks early.

Cervical cancer incidence peaks in midlife, with many cases diagnosed in women aged 50–60.

Women who have not undergone regular screenings earlier may have undetected pre-cancerous changes.

Menopause clinics often act as the first healthcare contact for women seeking advice on menopause-related issues, making it an ideal setting for routine cervical cancer screening.

Updated cervical cancer screening guidelines from **American Cancer Society (ACS)** recommend starting screening at age 25 with an HPV test and having HPV testing every 5 years through age 65. However, testing with an HPV/Pap co-test every 5 years or with a Pap test every 3 years is still acceptable. (17th May 2024).

Screening Methods

- **Pap Smear (Papanicolaou Test)**
  - Detects abnormal cervical cells (pre-cancerous or cancerous).
  - Recommended every 3 years for women aged 21–65.

- **HPV (Human Papillomavirus) Testing**
  - Identifies high-risk HPV types responsible for most cervical cancers.
  - Can be combined with a Pap smear (co-testing) every 5 years for women aged 30–65.

- **Visual Inspection with Acetic Acid (VIA)**
  - A cost-effective alternative in resource-limited settings.
  - Effective for identifying visible abnormalities on the cervix.

- **Colposcopy**
  - Follow-up procedure for women with abnormal Pap or HPV test results.

Screening for Postmenopausal Women:

- **Age Range**: Routine screening is recommended for women up to 65 years.

- **Discontinuation Criteria**: Women older than 65 may discontinue screening if:
  - They have had regular screenings in the past.
  - No history of cervical dysplasia or cancer.
  - **History of Hysterectomy**: Women who have had a total hysterectomy for non-cancerous reasons and no history of cervical dysplasia may not need screening.

2. Screening for Endometrial Cancer:

Importance of Endometrial Cancer Screening in Menopause Clinic

- Over 75% of uterine cancer cases occur in postmenopausal women.
- Risk factors like obesity, hormone therapy, diabetes, and unopposed estrogen make this population particularly vulnerable.
- Uterine cancer is often detected at an early stage due to symptoms like postmenopausal bleeding.
- Early diagnosis significantly improves survival rates and treatment outcome.
- Menopause clinics provide an ideal setting for evaluating symptoms, educating women about risks, and initiating timely diagnostic procedures.

Symptoms That Warrant Screening

- **Postmenopausal Bleeding**
  Any bleeding after menopause should be thoroughly investigated.
- **Unusual Vaginal Discharge**
  Watery, pink, or blood-tinged discharge may indicate malignancy.
- **Pelvic Pain or Pressure**
  Persistent discomfort or mass sensation should prompt further evaluation.

Risk Assessment in Menopause Clinics

Menopause clinics assess risk factors to identify women at higher risk of uterine cancer:

- **Unopposed Estrogen Use**
  Women on hormone replacement therapy without progesterone.

- **Obesity**
  Excess estrogen production from adipose tissue increases risk.

- **Family History**
  Lynch syndrome (hereditary nonpolyposis colorectal cancer) increases risk.

- **Medical History**
  Polycystic ovary syndrome (PCOS), diabetes, or hypertension.

Preventive Strategies

- **Weight Management**
  Reducing obesity through lifestyle counseling.

- **HRT Monitoring**
  Providing balanced hormone therapy to reduce endometrial cancer risk.

- **Regular Follow-Up**
  For women with risk factors or a history of atypical endometrial hyperplasia.

Screening Methods for Endometrial Cancer

Routine screening for endometrial cancer is not currently recommended for asymptomatic women. However, the following diagnostic evaluations are essential for those at risk or presenting symptoms:

- **Transvaginal Ultrasound (TVUS)**
  Evaluates the thickness of the endometrium.

- An **endometrial thickness >4 mm** in postmenopausal women raises suspicion and warrants further investigation.

- **Endometrial Biopsy**
  - **Gold standard for diagnosing endometrial cancer.**
  - Performed in women with postmenopausal bleeding or abnormal findings on ultrasound.

- **Hysteroscopy**
  Allows direct visualization of the uterine cavity and targeted biopsy of suspicious areas.

In summary, although routine uterine cancer screening for asymptomatic women is not recommended, menopause clinics play a pivotal role in early diagnosis and prevention through symptom evaluation, risk assessment, and targeted diagnostic interventions. These clinics empower women to take charge of their health during this critical phase of life, ensuring timely care and improving outcomes.

3. Screening for Ovarian Cancer

According to the current **International Guidelines**, routine ovarian cancer screening is not recommended for the general population due to lack of highly sensitive and specific screening tests.

The consensus among major medical organizations is in agreement with **United State Preventive Services Task Force**

(UNPSTF) that screening for ovarian cancer in the general population is not recommended.

Importance of Screening in Menopause Clinics

- Increased risk of ovarian cancer in postmenopausal women.
- Early detection can improve survival rates.
- Challenges in detecting ovarian cancer due to nonspecific symptoms.

Target Population

- **Asymptomatic Women:**
  - Routine risk assessment for all postmenopausal women.
- **High-Risk Women:**
  - Family history of ovarian or breast cancer.
  - BRCA1 or BRCA2 gene mutation carriers.
  - Personal history of other malignancies (e.g., breast or colon cancer).
- **Symptomatic Women:**
  - Persistent abdominal bloating, indigestion or nausea, changes in appetite, early satiety, pelvic pain/pressure, or urinary symptoms.

Screening Tools

- **Clinical Assessment**
  - Comprehensive medical and family history.
  - Physical examination (focus on abdominal and pelvic regions).

- **Imaging Techniques**
  - **Transvaginal Ultrasound (TVUS):**
    - Primary modality for detecting ovarian abnormalities.
    - Monitors size and morphology of ovarian masses.
  - **Doppler Ultrasound:**
    - Assess vascular flow to differentiate benign from malignant masses.

- **Biomarker Testing**
  - **CA-125 Levels:**
    - Useful in identifying malignancy, though not specific.
    - Serial measurements may improve predictive value.

  - **HE4 (Human Epididymis Protein 4):**
    - Combined with CA-125 for better specificity (e.g., Risk of Ovarian Malignancy Algorithm - ROMA).

- **Risk Prediction Models**
  - ROMA (Risk of Ovarian Malignancy Algorithm).
  - OVA1 (Multivariate index assay).
  - Risk models combining family history and genetic predisposition.

- **Genetic Testing and Counseling**
  - Offer BRCA1/2 testing to high-risk individuals.
  - Include comprehensive genetic counseling for those with positive findings.

- **Follow-Up and Referral**
  - Regular follow-up for women with benign findings.
  - Immediate referral to gynecologic oncologists for:
    - Persistent or enlarging masses.
    - Suspicious imaging or biomarker results.

- **Challenges and Limitations**
    - Lack of a universally accepted, cost-effective screening method.
    - Potential for false positives leading to unnecessary interventions.
    - Ethical considerations in asymptomatic populations.

- **Recommendations and Guidelines**
    - Follow national or international guidelines (e.g., ACOG, NCCN, FIGO).
    - Avoid routine screening in low-risk asymptomatic populations unless clinically indicated.

4. Breast Cancer Screening

Importance of Screening in Menopause Clinics

- Increased risk of breast cancer with advancing age and menopause.

- Early detection significantly improves prognosis and survival.

- Hormone replacement therapy (HRT) usage in menopause can influence breast cancer risk.

Target Population

- **Asymptomatic Women:**
    - All postmenopausal women as part of routine health check-ups.

- **High-Risk Women:**
    - Family history of breast or ovarian cancer.
    - Genetic predisposition (e.g., BRCA1/BRCA2 mutations).

    - Personal history of breast atypia or prior breast cancer.

- **Symptomatic Women:**
    - Presence of breast lump, nipple discharge, skin changes, or pain.

Screening Tools

- **Clinical Assessment**
    - Detailed history:
        - Family history of breast cancer.
        - History of HRT use or other risk factors.
    - Physical examination:
        - Palpation of breast tissue and axillary lymph nodes.
- **Imaging Techniques**
    - **Mammography:**
        - Primary screening tool for women aged 40 and above.
        - Digital mammography offers higher accuracy in postmenopausal women.
    - **Ultrasound:**
        - Supplemental tool for dense breast tissue or inconclusive mammography results.
    - **MRI:**
        - Recommended for high-risk women (e.g., BRCA mutation carriers) in conjunction with mammography.

Risk Assessment Models

- **Gail Model:**
    - Estimates 5-year and lifetime risk of breast cancer.

- **Tyrer-Cuzick Model:**
    - Incorporates family history and genetic predisposition.

    - Use risk calculators to stratify women into low, moderate, or high-risk groups.

- **Genetic Testing and Counseling**
    - BRCA1/2 testing for women with significant family history.

    - Provide genetic counseling to interpret results and plan personalized screening.

- **Screening Intervals**
    - **Average-Risk Women:**
        - Mammography every 1-2 years starting at age 40-50, continuing until at least 74.

    - **High-Risk Women:**
        - Annual mammography and MRI starting at an earlier age based on guidelines.
        - Tailor screening intervals based on clinical and genetic risk factors.

- **Lifestyle and Preventive Strategies**
    - Encourage lifestyle modifications:
        - Regular exercise.
        - Healthy diet.
        - Limiting alcohol consumption.

    - Discuss risk reduction strategies:
        - Chemoprevention for high-risk women (e.g., tamoxifen, raloxifene).
        - Prophylactic mastectomy in extreme high-risk cases (BRCA-positive).

- **Follow-Up and Referral**
    - Monitor findings from routine screening.

- Refer to a breast specialist or oncologist for:
    - Suspicious imaging findings.
    - Palpable masses or changes requiring biopsy.
    - Management of high-risk women.

- **Challenges and Limitations**
  - Overdiagnosis and false positives from mammography.

  - Anxiety associated with screening in low-risk populations.

  - Variability in adherence to screening guidelines.

- **Recommendations and Guidelines**
  - Adhere to established guidelines (e.g., ACOG, USPSTF, NCCN).

  - Individualize screening plans based on patient preferences and risk profile.

CHAPTER IV: UNDERSTANDING MENOPAUSE HORMONE THERAPY (MHT)

"Medicine is not only a science;

it is also an art of letting our patients embrace hope."

– Anonymous

(A) Definition of MHT

Menopause Hormone Therapy (MHT), also known as Hormone Replacement Therapy (HRT), is a medical treatment that involves the administration of hormones, primarily estrogen and progestogen (or progesterone), to alleviate symptoms associated with menopause. MHT is designed to replenish hormone levels that naturally decline during menopause, aiming to improve quality of life and manage health risks associated with hormonal changes.

Usefulness of MHT

- **Relief from Menopausal Symptoms**:
  - Reduces **hot flashes**, **night sweats**, and **vaginal dryness**.
  - Improves **sleep disturbances** caused by menopausal symptoms.
  - Helps manage **mood swings**, anxiety, and irritability.

- **Bone Health**:
  - Reduces the risk of **osteoporosis** by maintaining bone density.
  - Lowers the likelihood of **fractures**, particularly in postmenopausal women.

- **Cardiovascular Health** (in early postmenopause):
    - May improve cholesterol levels and reduce the risk of heart disease if initiated early in menopause.

- **Cognitive and Mental Health**:
    - Potentially reduces the risk of **cognitive decline** and may alleviate symptoms of mild depression.

- **Urogenital Health**:
    - Improves **urinary symptoms** like frequency and urgency.
    - Enhances **sexual health** by addressing discomfort during intercourse.

- **Quality of Life**:
    - Overall improvement in physical and emotional well-being by alleviating symptoms that interfere with daily activities.

Considerations

- The benefits of MHT vary based on the individual's age, timing of initiation, and specific health conditions.

- MHT should be personalized and prescribed after a thorough evaluation of risks and benefits by a healthcare provider.

Terminologies in Relation to Menopause

- **MHT**: Menopause Hormone Therapy
- **HRT**: Hormone Replacement Therapy
- **HT**: Hormone Therapy
- **ET**: Estrogen Therapy
- **EPT**: Estrogen-Progesterone Therapy
- **AT:** Androgen Therapy
- **SERM**: Selective Estrogen Receptor Modulator (e.g. Ospemifene, Raloxifene)

- **TSEC**: Tissue Selective Estrogen Compound (e.g. Bazedoxifene)
- **STEAR**: Selective Tissue Estrogen Activity Regulator (e.g. Tibolone)

(B) Understanding Estrogen

Estrogen is largely responsible for the development and maintenance of the female reproductive system, secondary sexual characters and have also an effect on nonreproductive systems. Endogenous estrogens are available in various forms, the concentration of which depends on the stage of a woman's life.

Endogenous Estrogen:

Here's a systematic enumeration of **endogenous estrogens—E1 (Estrone), E2 (Estradiol), E3 (Estriol)**, and **E4 (Estetrol)**—covering their availability, potency, synthesis, and bioavailability across different stages of a woman's life:

Chemical Structure of Estrogen:

Major Circulating Estrogens In Women

Three major naturally occurring circulating estrogens in women:

•Estrone (E1)

•Estradiol (E2) most potent

•Estriol (E3) least potent

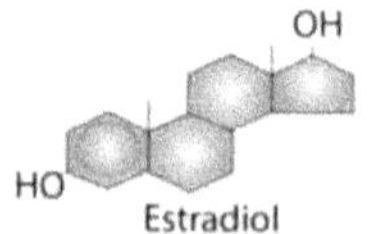

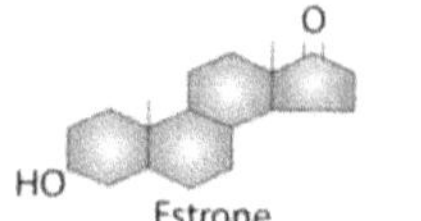

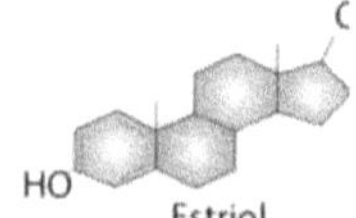

1. Estrone (E1)

- **Potency**:
  - Moderate estrogenic activity; less potent than estradiol (E2).

- **Synthesis**:
  - Predominantly synthesized in adipose tissue via **aromatization of androstenedione**.

  - Major estrogen during **postmenopause**.

- **Availability in Life Stages**:
  - **Reproductive years**: Present in low concentrations.

  - **Menopause**: Dominant estrogen due to peripheral conversion in adipose tissue.

- **Bioavailability**:
  - Moderate systemic bioavailability as it circulates bound to sex hormone-binding globulin (SHBG) and albumin.

  - Longer half-life compared to E2.

2. Estradiol (E2)

- **Potency**:
  - The most potent natural estrogen.

- **Synthesis**:
  - Synthesized primarily in the **ovarian follicles** from testosterone via aromatase during the reproductive years.

- In **pre-menopause**, E2 is the dominant estrogen.

- Declines significantly in menopause; minimal synthesis occurs in peripheral tissues.

- **Availability in Life Stages**:
  - **Childhood**: Minimal levels.

  - **Reproductive years**: Dominant estrogen; peaks during follicular and luteal phases of the menstrual cycle.

  - **Menopause**: Declines significantly; minimal residual synthesis occurs.

- **Bioavailability**:
  - Highly bioavailable during reproductive years.

  - Circulates bound to SHBG and albumin; free E2 is biologically active.

  - Short half-life compared to E1 but metabolically active.

3. Estriol (E3)

- **Potency**:
  - Weakest estrogen.

- **Synthesis**:
  - Produced in significant amounts during **pregnancy**.

  - Synthesized in the placenta from **16α-hydroxy dehydroepiandrosterone sulfate (16α-OH DHEAS)**, a fetal adrenal precursor.

- **Availability in Life Stages**:
  - **Non-pregnant state**: Minimal levels; formed as a metabolite of E2 and E1 in the liver.

- **Pregnancy**: Becomes the predominant estrogen, especially in the third trimester.

- **Bioavailability**:
  - Weak systemic estrogenic effects due to low receptor affinity.
  - Rapid metabolism and clearance.

4. Estetrol (E4)

Another type of oestrogen called **Estetrol (E4)** was discovered by **Dicxtolus in 1965, produced exclusively from foetal liver during pregnancy.** It is not convertible to E2, E3. Lots of trials were being conducted since then for its potential use in hormone therapy and contraception. It is already introduced in combined contraceptive pills with progesterone. Its use as hormone therapy is under study.

It is considered the fourth major endogenous estrogen, alongside estrone (E1), estradiol (E2), and estriol (E3).

- **Biochemical Characteristics**
  - **Molecular Formula**: $C_{18}H_{24}O_4$.
  - **Structure**: Estetrol has four hydroxyl groups, which make it distinct from other estrogens.
  - **Lipophilicity**: Lower compared to estradiol, resulting in a different pharmacokinetic profile.
  - **Binding**: Selectively binds to estrogen receptors (ERα and ERβ), but with weaker affinity compared to estradiol.

- **Physiological Role**
  - Synthesized by the fetal liver from precursors produced by the placenta - from 15α-hydroxy dehydroepiandrosterone sulfate (15α-OH DHEAS).

  - Peaks in maternal and fetal circulation during the third trimester of pregnancy.

  - Functions as a biomarker for fetal well-being and placental health.

  - Non-pregnant state: Absent post-delivery.

- **Pharmacological Properties**
  - **Selective Estrogen Receptor Modulator (SERM)-** like activity: Exhibits tissue-specific estrogenic effects.

  - **Half-Life**: Longer compared to estradiol and estriol, enabling sustained action.

  - **Oral Bioavailability**: High, making it suitable for therapeutic use.

  - **Metabolism**: Primarily metabolized by the liver.

- **Clinical Applications (Potential Therapeutic Use)**
  - Hormone replacement therapy (HRT) during menopause due to its favorable safety profile. Not yet introduced in hormone therapy, lots of studies and experimental trials are going on.

  - Contraceptive applications, often combined with progestins. The preparation is already available in market.

- **Safety Profile**:
  - Low risk of stimulating breast and endometrial tissues compared to estradiol.

- **Neuroprotective Effects**:
  - Being studied for its potential protective role in cognitive functions.

- **Comparative Distinction**
  - **From Estradiol (E2)**: Lower potency but more selective action, leading to reduced side effects.

  - **From Estriol (E3)**: Longer half-life and more sustained activity.

  - **From Estrone (E1)**: Predominantly produced in pregnancy and not in postmenopausal women.

- **Research and Development**
  - Active area of investigation for its use in:
    - ✓ Safer contraceptives.

    - ✓ Menopause-related therapies.

Summary of Synthesis and Role by Stage

Stage	**Dominant Estrogen**	**Source of Synthesis**	**Role**
Childhood	Minimal	Peripheral Conversion	Limited biological role
Reproductive Years	Estradiol (E2)	Ovaries	Regulates Menstrual Cycle
Pregnancy	Estriol (E3), Estetrol (E4)	Placenta (E3), Fetal liver (E4)	Fetal development and maternal adaptation
Postmenopause	Estrone (E1)	Adipose tissue	Maintains minimal estrogenic effects

Relative Potency of Estrogens (E2 > E1 > E3 > E4)

- **Estradiol (E2)** is the most potent, with significant systemic and local actions on tissues.
- **Estrone (E1)** has moderate potency, mainly postmenopausal significance.
- **Estriol (E3)** and **Estetrol (E4)** are weaker, with specific roles during pregnancy.

Estrogen Receptor Distribution and Regulation in the Female Body

Estrogen plays a pivotal role in regulating various physiological processes in the female body. Its effects are mediated through two main types of estrogen receptors (ERs): **ERα (Estrogen Receptor Alpha)** and **ERβ (Estrogen Receptor Beta)**. These receptors are distributed in different tissues and are subject to complex regulatory mechanisms.

Estrogen Receptors

Estrogen Target Tissues

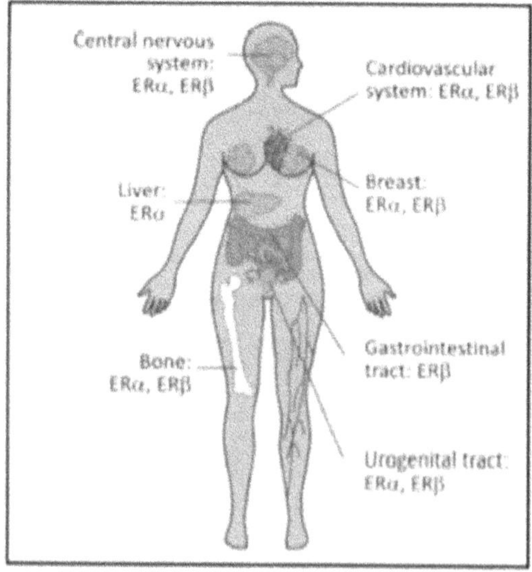

Tissue Distribution

- **Reproductive System**
  - **Uterus**: High concentration of ERα, regulating uterine growth, endometrial proliferation, and preparation for pregnancy.
  - **Ovaries**: Both ERα and ERβ, important for follicular development and ovulation.
  - **Mammary Glands**: Predominantly ERα, involved in ductal development and lactation preparation.
  - **Vagina**: ERα influences epithelial integrity and lubrication.
- **Skeletal System**
  - ERα: Critical for bone remodeling and maintaining bone density by regulating osteoblast and osteoclast activity.
- **Cardiovascular System**
  - Both ERα and ERβ: Protect against atherosclerosis by modulating lipid metabolism and promoting vasodilation through nitric oxide production.
- **Nervous System**
  - ERβ: Neuroprotective effects, influencing mood, cognition, and memory.
  - ERα: Regulates hypothalamic function, controlling reproductive hormone release and thermoregulation.
- **Immune System**
  - ERβ: Modulates inflammation and immune responses by influencing cytokine production and immune cell activity.

ER- alpha and ER-beta exhibit distinct as well overlapping functions at the level of DNA binding. Nuclear and membrane ER are biochemically identical.

Exogenous Estrogen:

Mainly of two types:

1.Natural Estrogen 2. Synthetic Estrogen

1. Natural Estrogen:

Natural estrogen is used for MHT.

- **Oral Route** – Most commonly used route in the form of tablets.
    - 17 Beta Estradiol
    - Estradiol valerate
    - Estriol
    - Conjugated Equine Oestrogen (CEE)
        - ✓ Derived from natural sources (pregnant mare's urine).
        - ✓ Contains a mix of estrone sulfate, equilin sulfate, and other estrogenic compounds.
        - ✓ Long history of use in HRT.
        - ✓ 0.625 mg of CEE corresponds to 2 mg of oral estradiol and 50 mcg of transdermal estradiol.
        - ✓ Appears to be equally effective for hot flashes.

17 beta estradiol is preferred over other estrogens, because it is structurally identical with the endogenous estrogen secreted by the ovaries.

- **Transdermal Route:**
  Used in special situations, in the form of patches, gel or spray, where oral route is contraindicated.
    - 17 beta estradiol
    - Conjugated Equine Estrogen (CEE)

- **Vaginal Route:**
  Exclusively used for Genitourinary Syndrome of Menopause (GSM) in the form of creams, tablets and vaginal rings.
    - Estriol
    - CEE
    - 17 beta estradiol

Doses of Estrogen used in MHT

Estrogen	Ultralow dose	Low dose	Standard dose	High dose
Oral CEE	0.15 mg	0.3 – 0.45 mg	0.625 mg	1.25 mg
Oral 17 beta estradiol	0.5 mg	1 mg	2 mg	4 mg
Oral estradiol valerate	0.5 mg	1 mg	2 mg	-
Transdermal 17beta estradiol	14 mcg	25 mcg	50 mcg	100 mcg

Oral vs Transdermal Route

Oral Route:

- Convenient daily dosing.

- Orally administered naturally occurring oestrogens are rapidly metabolised in both gut and liver through a metabolic process called "**first pass effect**". Hence a larger effective dose is needed.

- Hepatic effect with oral ET results in:
    - Increased Triglycerides
    - Increased SHBG

- Increased C-Reactive Proteins
- Increased Clotting Factors
- Increased HDL-C and decreased LDL-C

- May have nausea and more tendency for weight gain due to fluid retention, breast tenderness especially initially.
- May cause an increase in VTE risk.

Transdermal Route:

- Convenient weekly/twice weekly dosing if using patch and daily if using gel.
- As it avoids the "**first pass effect**", a much lower effective dose is required. Dose is delivered directly into the bloodstream.
- Less tendency for weight gain / breast tenderness.
- Decrease LDL-C but no change in HDL-C.
- No change or decrease in triglycerides.
- No change in inflammatory markers.
- No increased risk in VTE.

Transdermal route preferred over oral route in women with:

- Hypertriglyceridemia (> 500 mg/dl)
- BMI > 30
- Personal/ Family history of VTE
- Thrombophilia

- Moderate/Severe risk of CVD
- Gallbladder disease
- Migraine headaches with aura
- Varicose veins

Factors Affecting Oral Estrogen Metabolism and Their Clinical Implications

- **Medications Affecting Oral Estrogen Metabolism:**
  - **Inducers of Estrogen Metabolism**
    These medications increase CYP450 enzyme activity, accelerating estrogen breakdown and reducing efficacy.
    - ✓ **Anticonvulsants**:
      Phenytoin, Carbamazepine, Phenobarbital
    - ✓ **Antimicrobials**:
      Rifampin (antibiotic), Griseofulvin (antifungal)
  - **Inhibitors of Estrogen Metabolism:**
    These medications inhibit CYP450 enzymes, slowing estrogen metabolism and increasing systemic levels, which may heighten the risk of side effects.
    - ✓ **Antifungal Agents**:
      Ketoconazole, Itraconazole
    - ✓ **Macrolide Antibiotics**:
      Erythromycin, Clarithromycin
    - ✓ **Calcium Channel Blockers**:
      Diltiazem, Verapamil
  - **Medications Affecting Enterohepatic Circulation**
    These medications reduce reabsorption of estrogens in the intestines, decreasing circulating levels.
    - ✓ **Antibiotics**:
      Broad-spectrum antibiotics disrupt gut flora, reducing enterohepatic recycling.

- ✓ **Bile Acid Sequestrants**:
  Cholestyramine binds estrogens in the gut, reducing reabsorption.

- o **Other Interacting Medications**
  - ✓ **Thyroid Hormones**:
    High doses can accelerate estrogen metabolism by increasing hepatic enzyme activity. Oral oestrogen increases thyroid binding globulin (TBG) which results in low bioavailability of thyroxine and hence may have to increase thyroxine dose in a woman with hypothyroidism. Can be easily tracked with thyroid stimulating hormone (TSH) level.

- **Body Composition**
  - o **Body Fat**:
    Estrogens are lipophilic and can accumulate in adipose tissue, potentially affecting metabolism and bioavailability in obese individuals.

Clinical Implications

- o **Reduced Efficacy**:
  Enzyme inducers may lead to inadequate symptom relief or increased risk of breakthrough menopausal symptoms.

- o **Increased Side Effects**:
  Enzyme inhibitors may elevate estrogen levels, causing nausea, breast tenderness, or thromboembolic events.

- o **Monitoring and Adjustments**:
  - ✓ Dose adjustments may be required based on interacting medications.
  - ✓ Switching to non-oral routes (transdermal, vaginal) bypasses first-pass metabolism and minimizes interactions.

2. Synthetic Estrogen:

Ethinyl Estradiol

It is not used for MHT.

It is used in contraceptives.

It is 750 – 1000 times more potent than natural estrogens.

(C) Understanding Progesterone used in MHT:

Progesterone plays a critical role in Menopause Hormone Therapy (MHT) as it helps mitigate the risks associated with unopposed estrogen therapy, particularly for women with an intact uterus. Below is a systematic explanation of its role, benefits, types, and clinical considerations.

Overview of Progesterone in MHT

- **Purpose**: Progesterone is primarily used in MHT to prevent **endometrial hyperplasia** and **endometrial cancer**, which can occur due to the proliferative effects of estrogen on the uterine lining.

- **Mechanism**: Progesterone counterbalances the effect of estrogen by inducing secretory changes in the endometrium and promoting cellular turnover, thus reducing the risk of abnormal cell growth.

- **Indications for Use**
  - **Women with an intact uterus**: Progesterone is always included in the regimen if estrogen therapy is prescribed.

  - **Hysterectomised women with history of endometriosis.**

  - **Women who have undergone subtotal hysterectomy.** Unopposed oestrogen may stimulate the remnant pathology and hence in such cases also progesterone needs to be supplemented.

- **Forms of Progesterone Used in MHT**
  Progesterone in MHT is available in various forms, each with specific indications and advantages:

- **Natural Micronized Progesterone (NMP)**:
  - ✓ **Description**: Biologically identical to endogenous progesterone.
  - ✓ **Advantages**:
    - Better safety profile.
    - Fewer side effects on lipids and coagulation.
  - ✓ **Usage**: Often used orally or vaginally.
- **Dydrogesterone:**
  - ✓ **Structure and Function**:
    - A retro-progesterone structurally similar to natural progesterone.
    - Exhibits high selectivity for progesterone receptors.
    - Lacks androgenic, glucocorticoid, and mineralocorticoid activity, making it more tolerable for patients.
  - ✓ **Favorable Safety Profile**:
    - Minimal side effects compared to synthetic progestins like medroxyprogesterone acetate (MPA).
    - Does not negatively impact lipid metabolism or glucose tolerance.
  - ✓ **Forms and Administration**
    Oral Formulation:
    - Dydrogesterone is commonly available in oral form.
    - Easy to administer and well-tolerated.
- **Synthetic Progestins**:
  - ✓ **Examples**: Medroxyprogesterone acetate (MPA), norethisterone, levonorgestrel.
  - ✓ **Advantages**:
    - Stronger progestogenic effect.

- Long-acting formulations available.

✓ **Disadvantages**:
Higher risk of cardiovascular side effects and breast cancer compared to NMP.

- **Local Progesterone Delivery (Intrauterine Devices – IUDs)**: **e.g.** Levonorgestrel-releasing intrauterine system (LNG-IUS).

✓ **Advantages**:
- Direct endometrial effect with minimal systemic absorption.
- Reduces abnormal uterine bleeding and can treat endometrial hyperplasia.

Right progesterone molecule, as a component of MHT, always makes a difference.

Micronized progesterone (natural progesterone) and Dydrogesterone (retro-progesterone) appear to be the safest option, with lower associated risk in relation to cardiovascular, thromboembolic and breast cancer compared with other synthetic progestogens.

Also micronized progesterone and dydrogesterone are the first-choice options for use in special situations such as in women with high density breast tissue, diabetes, obesity, smoking and risk factors for thromboembolism.

The structure of natural micronized progesterone is closer to the endogenous progesterone and is obtained primarily from plant sources. They are currently available in oral, vaginal and injectable formulations.

Progesterone exhibits its pregestational activity by binding nuclear progesterone receptors (PR) and by interacting with membrane progesterone receptors (mPR).

Drospirenone, a derivative of 17-spironolactone, acts on mineralocorticoid receptors to prevent sodium retention and thus reduces estrogen related sodium and water. It maintains HDL-C and triglyceride levels, lowers blood pressure in hypertensive women, therefore a preferred choice in postmenopausal women with hypertension.

Comparison Between Micronized Progesterone, Dydrogesterone and MPA

Parameters	Micronized Progesterone	Dydrogesterone	MPA
Structure	Identical to natural Progesterone	Structurally similar to natural progesterone	Synthetic Derivative of progesterone
Endometrial Protection	Highly Effective	Highly Effective	Highly Effective
Breast Cancer Risk	Neutral to minimal	Lower risk compared to MPA	Slightly increased risk with long term use
Cardiovascular Impact	Neutral to favourable	Neutral to favourable	Associated with higher thromboembolic and CVD risk.
Lipid Profile Impact	Neutral to favourable	Neutral	Increases LDL and decreases HDL
Metabolic Effects	Neutral	Neutral to Positive	Negative impact on lipid and glucose metabolism

Micronized progesterone and dydrogesterone are preferred in MHT due to their superior safety profiles, favorable impact on cardiovascular and metabolic health, and better tolerability compared to synthetic progestins like medroxyprogesterone acetate. Individualized therapy should consider patient-specific risks and preferences.

Progesterone and their dosages in sequential combined regimen of MHT:

For sequential combined MHT, the progesterone phase should be at least 10 days and preferably 12-14 days per cycle to provide sufficient endometrial protection.

Progesterone	**Route**	**Low dose**	**High dose**
Micronized progesterone	Oral	100 mg	200 mg
Dydrogesterone	Oral	5 mg	10 mg

(D) Patient Selection for MHT:

Hormone therapy is most often used to treat common menopausal symptoms including hot flashes and vaginal discomfort.

Hormone therapy has also been proved to prevent bone loss and reduce fractures in postmenopausal women.

However, there are risks associated with using hormone therapy. These risks depend on the type of hormone therapy, the dose, the duration and individual health risks. For best results, hormone therapy should be tailored to individual women and re-evaluated now and then to be sure that **benefits far outweigh the risk**.

Basic types of hormone therapy:

Menopausal hormone therapy primarily focuses on replacing the estrogen that ovaries no longer secrete after menopause. There are two main types of hormone therapies.

Systemic hormone therapy:

The primary goal of systemic MHT is to relieve hot flashes. The other symptoms associated with perimenopause and postmenopause that respond to hormone therapy include sleep disturbances, mood swings, depression and in some cases joint aches and pains.

Low dose vaginal estrogen therapy:

Low dose vaginal preparations of estrogen which either comes in cream, tablet and ring forms; minimize the amount of estrogen absorbed and therefore avoiding systemic side effects. These preparations are exclusively used to treat the genitourinary system of menopause.

In women with both vasomotor and genitourinary symptoms, both systemic and vaginal estrogen therapy can be started, if needed.

Updated Clinical Guidelines on MHT:

Besides detailed history, physical examination and recommended investigations, the following 5 factors do play a major role in selecting patients for MHT.

1.Age of patient
2.Severity of symptoms
3.Calculating risk factors for CVD and breast cancer.
4.Selection of estrogen/progesterone, doses and duration of therapy.
5.Accessibility of therapy.

1. Age of the patient:

- Age of the patient is the major determinant of the risks and benefits of MHT.

- MHT initiated within 10 years of menopause and below 60 years of age for menopausal symptoms in healthy menopausal women:
    - ✓ Reduces the risk of all-cause mortality and Cardiovascular Disease Risk compared with placebo or no treatment.

    - ✓ Cochrane Collaborative Review reported 30 % related risk reductions.

    - ✓ Benefits always outweigh the risks.

"Timings of MHT are always a window of opportunity".

(Timing Hypothesis)

- **Age < 50 years of age:**
  Benefits far outweigh the risks.
  MHT should be offered to symptomatic women.

- **Age 50 – 60 years of age:**
  Benefits outweigh the risks.
  MHT should be offered.

- **Age > 60 years of age:**
  Risks outweigh the benefit
  Treatment should be avoided or individualised.

2. Severity of symptoms:

- Vasomotor symptoms are the most common indication for the use of MHT.

- ***Women with mild symptoms do not need hormone therapy. Mild symptoms can be relieved with lifestyle modifications and counselling.***

- The majority of women with moderate to severe symptoms associated with a negative impact on sleep and quality of life, are the candidates for MHT.

- **Menopause Rating Scale (MRS)** is a standardized tool to assess the menopausal symptoms. It has been widely used to assess the symptoms of menopause and their severity in the population worldwide.

- MRS is a health-related quality of life scale (HRQoL) and was developed in response to the lack of standardized scale to measure the severity of aging symptoms and their impact on the HRQoL in early 1990.

Menopause Rating Scale (MRS):

The **Menopause Rating Scale (MRS)** is a widely used tool to evaluate the severity of menopause-related symptoms. It consists of three domains: **somatic**, **psychological**, and **urogenital**, with a total of 11 symptoms. Below is a systematic enumeration:

Menopause Rating Scale (MRS)

Which of the following symptoms apply to you at this time?

(X ONE Box For EACH Symptom) For Symptoms That Do Not Apply, Please Mark "None").

Symptoms:	none	mild	moderate	severe	extremely severe
Score	= 0	1	2	3	4
1. Hot flashes, sweating (episodes of sweating)	☐	☐	☐	☐	☐
2. Heart discomfort (unusual awareness of heart beat, heart skipping, heart racing, tightness)	☐	☐	☐	☐	☐
3. Sleep problems (difficulty in falling asleep, difficulty in sleeping through the night, waking up early)	☐	☐	☐	☐	☐
4. Depressive mood (feeling down, sad, on the verge of tears, lack of drive, mood swings)	☐	☐	☐	☐	☐
5. Irritability (feeling nervous, inner tension, feeling aggressive)	☐	☐	☐	☐	☐
6. Anxiety (inner restlessness, feeling panicky)	☐	☐	☐	☐	☐
7. Physical and mental exhaustion (general decrease in performance, impaired memory, decrease in concentration, forgetfulness)	☐	☐	☐	☐	☐
8. Sexual problems (change in sexual desire, in sexual activity and satisfaction)	☐	☐	☐	☐	☐
9. Bladder problems (difficulty in urinating, increased need to urinate, bladder incontinence)	☐	☐	☐	☐	☐
10. Dryness of vagina (sensation of dryness or burning in the vagina, difficulty with sexual intercourse)	☐	☐	☐	☐	☐
11. Joint and muscular discomfort (pain in the joints, rheumatoid complaints)	☐	☐	☐	☐	☐

- According to **WHO** standard, the degree of severity is consistent with: None: 0, Mild: 1, Moderate: 2, Severe: 3, Very severe: 4.

- **Severity Classification Based on MRS Score:**

    - **0 to 4**: No or minimal symptoms.
    - **5 to 8**: Mild symptoms
    - **9 to 16**: Moderate symptoms
    - **17 to 44**: Severe symptoms

- Document the degree of symptomatology in terms of their severity/score on the menopause proforma for assessing the severity of symptoms, follow-up and effectiveness of the treatment.

- The scoring helps in assessing the impact of menopausal symptoms on quality of life and guides treatment or interventions.

  Source: *Heinemann LAJ, Potthoff P, Schneider HPG. International versions of MRS Health Quality of Life outcomes. 2003:1: 28.doi:10.1186/1477-7525-1-28.*

3. Calculating the Risk of Breast Cancer

Breast Cancer Risk Assessment Tool **(BCRAT)** also known as **Gail Model (*Gail et al., 1989; Claus et al., Constantine et al. 1999*).**

Breast cancer is among the most prevalent cancers that affect women, with more than 2 million fresh cases diagnosed each year worldwide.

Gail Model, an online calculator allows health providers to estimate a woman's risk of developing invasive breast cancer over the next 5 years and up to the age of 90 years (life time risk).

The Gail Model incorporates 6 breast cancer risks as follows:

- Age
- Age at Menarche
- Age at first live birth (or not given birth)
- Number of breast biopsies.
- Number of breast biopsies showing atypical hyperplasia
- Number of first-degree relatives with breast cancer (mother, sister or daughter).

Breast Cancer Risk Cut-offs for counselling before recommending MHT:

Risk Categories	5 yrs NCI or NBIS Breast Cancer Risk Assessment %	Suggested Approach
Low	< 1.67	MHT is ok
Moderate	1.67– 5	Transdermal route preferred
High	>5	Avoid MHT

NCI: National Cancer Institute, **IBIS:** International Breast Interventional Study, **MHT:** Menopause Hormone Therapy

Calculating the Risk of Cardiovascular Disease

Endocrine Society 2015 clinical guidelines suggest calculating Cardiovascular Disease Risk and Breast Cancer Risk before initiating MHT.

- World Health Organization / International Society of Hypertension (WHO/ISH) Risk Prediction Charts predict 10 years risk of combined myocardial infarction and stroke risk, fatal and nonfatal.

- Charts are useful for stratifying risk for people with blood pressure <160/100 mm of Hg or blood cholesterol < 8mmol/L or uncomplicated diabetes with or without treatment.
- In 2007, WHO/ISH published a series of 14 WHO sub regions risk prediction charts, each dedicated to different ethnic-geographic regions for south-east Asia.

- The risk factors affect the population group differently based on differences in the geographical location, resulting in significant variability in the absolute risk predicted by the major risk factors.

- Hard copies of CVD risk assessment charts can be downloaded from www.jmidlifehealth.org.

- Patient's Data is Required: Age, Sex, Total Cholesterol, Systolic Blood Pressure, Smoking status, Diabetic status, Hypertensive treatment.

CVD Risk Assessment

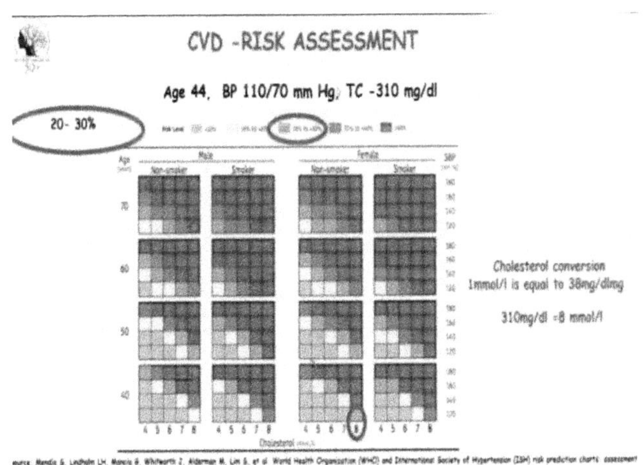

Recommendations of MHT according to the risk:

- **Low risk for CVD:** MHT safe in women
- **Moderate risk for CVD:** Prefer transdermal
- **High risk** for **CVD:** Avoid MHT

WHO/ISH Chart limitations:

- Obesity
- Family history of coronary heart disease or stroke in first degree relatives. (male < 55 yrs., female < 65 yrs.).
- Raised triglyceride level.
- Low HDL-C level (< 40 mg/dl).
- Raised levels of C - reactive protein, fibrinogen, homocysteine.
- Sedentary lifestyle.

And hence, may lead to underestimation of CVD risk.

Assessment of Baseline Risk for VTE:

High Risk – Avoid MHT

- Women with personal history of VTE.
- Women with first- or second-degree relatives with VTE.
- Inherited Thrombophilia.

Comparatively Low Risk – Prefer transdermal route or Tibolone

- Rising age
- Obesity
- Sedentary lifestyle
- Varicose veins

4. Selection of Estrogen / Progesterone, Dosages, and Duration

Preferred Estrogen and doses:

- Estrogen preferred is usually 17 beta Estradiol.

- Lower dosages started initially (oral 0.5 mg or transdermal 25 mcg) and titrated to relieve the symptoms.

- Relief from hot flashes often occurs within the first 3-4 weeks of therapy.

- If the patient has persistent hot flashes after 4th week, then the dose of estrogen is increased making it a standard dose.

- In women with premature ovarian insufficiency (POI), estrogen therapy needs to be initiated with a standard dose.

Preferred Progesterone and dose:

- Progesterone preferred is usually micronized progesterone or dydrogesterone.

- Studies showed that risk of invasive breast cancer was significantly lower with MHT containing either micronized progesterone or dydrogesterone than with MHT containing other progesterone such as MPA.

- Micronized progesterone dose 100 - 200 mg/day for sequential combined and 100 mg/day for continuous combined regimen.

- Dydrogesterone 5-10 mg/day for sequential combined and 5 mg/day for continuous combined regimen.

- For sequential combined MHT, the progesterone phase should be preferably 12-14 days per cycle to provide sufficient endometrial protection.

Duration of MHT use:

- Safety data of estrogen- progesterone therapy is 3 - 5 years while estrogen only therapy safety data for use is 7 years with a 20 years follow-up.

- Both **North American Menopause Society and the American College of Obstetrics & Gynaecology** recommend extended use of therapy in case of recurrence of symptoms after stoppage of therapy, but only after explaining the patients the risk and benefits.

- In premature ovarian failure (POI), MHT should be continued till the natural age of menopause and thereafter may be continued if the patient is symptomatic and there are no other contraindications for MHT: a shared decision between the patient and the gynaecologist.

Stop treatment:

- If migraine appears for the first time or if the headache gets worsened.

- Blurring of vision or any symptom suggestive of vascular occlusion.

- If jaundice appears.

- MHT is to be stopped 4-6 weeks before elective surgery.

Follow-up:

- Review after one month for efficacy and side effects. Check weight and blood pressure.

- After 3 months to access compliance. Check weight and blood pressure.

- Annually, include physical examination, update of medical and family history, relevant laboratory and imaging investigations, discussion on lifestyle, strategies to prevent age-related chronic diseases.

Different Regimens of MHT:

1. Combined MHT (E+P) Regimen

- Sequential combined
- Continuous combined

2. Estrogen only MHT (E) Regimen

Sequential Combined Regimen:

- Recommended in perimenopausal women.
- Estrogen daily for 28 days + Progesterone daily for last 14 days with hormone free interval of 3-6 days.
- 85-90 % of women receiving sequential combined regimen have monthly withdrawal bleeding.

Continuous Combined:

- Recommended in postmenopausal women.
- Estrogen + Progesterone for all days without break.
- Induces amenorrhoea in most women. Daily progesterone without break causes atrophic endometrium.

Estrogen only Regimen:

Recommended in hysterectomized women without break.

5. Accessibility of Therapy

Women in low and middle-income countries have limited or no access to MHT. In some countries there are few or no menopause clinics. Even, where the MHT is available, expertise is often lacking to prescribe it effectively, safely and ethically.

The International Menopause Society (established in 1970) in collaboration with the World Health Organization (WHO) has designated **October 18 as 'World Menopause Day' and month as 'Menopause Awareness Month.'** The global initiatives are dedicated to millions of mature women of 40 plus who are going to spend one-third of their life after menopause and are unaware or ignorant about the positive steps to be taken for improving their quality of life in the second inning.... **the postmenopausal life.**

Indian Menopause Society (established in 1995) with its member societies are trying hard to sensitize the healthcare providers especially the practicing gynecologists towards the health of menopausal women in promoting the concept of menopausal clinics all over India.

Few Words About Compounded Bioidentical MHT

Scientific statement by the **Endocrine Society and National Academics of Science, Medicine and Engineering** found that there was no rational for routine prescribing of unregulated, untested and potentially harmful custom compounded bioidentical hormone therapies, though these unlicenced preparations are marketed in some countries.

How is MHT Given?

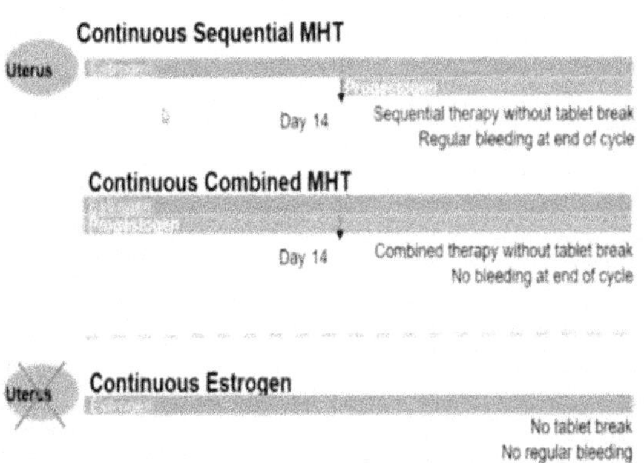

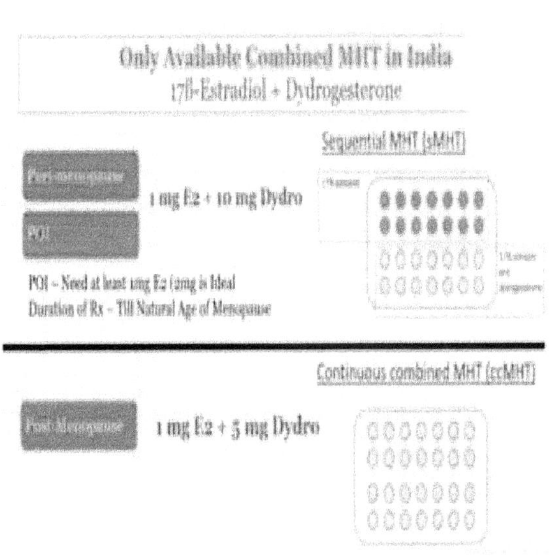

(F) Contraindications for MHT

Menopause Hormone Therapy (MHT) is highly effective in managing menopausal symptoms but must be prescribed cautiously. Certain medical conditions can increase the risk of complications, making MHT contraindicated in some cases. Below is a systematic list of absolute and relative contraindications:

Absolute Contraindications:

These are conditions where MHT should not be prescribed due to a high risk of adverse outcomes.

- **Hormone-Sensitive Cancers**:
  - Known, suspected, or history of **breast cancer**.
  - Known, suspected, or history of **endometrial cancer**.
- **Unexplained Vaginal Bleeding**:
  - Undiagnosed abnormal genital bleeding, which could indicate underlying malignancy.
- **Active or History of Venous Thromboembolism (VTE)**:
  - Deep vein thrombosis (DVT).
  - Pulmonary embolism (PE).
- **Active or History of Arterial Thromboembolic Events**:
  - Stroke.
  - Myocardial infarction (heart attack).
- **Liver Disease**:
  - Active liver dysfunction or disease (e.g., hepatitis, cirrhosis) since hormones are metabolized in the liver.
- **Known or Suspected Pregnancy**:
  - Hormone therapy is contraindicated during pregnancy.
- **Active Gall Bladder Disease:**

CHAPTER V: MANAGING VASOMOTOR SYMPTOMS

"Health is a state of complete harmony

of the body, mind, and spirit.

When one is free from physical disabilities

and mental distractions, the gates of the soul open."

– B.K.S. Iyengar

(A) Key points:

- VMS or hot flashes and night sweats are often considered the cardinal symptoms of menopause. VMS are episodes of profuse heat accompanied by sweating and flashing, experienced predominantly around the head, neck, chest and upper back.

- The incidence increases typically during perimenopause. The transition period begins almost 3-4 years before the occurrence of menopause. As this transition period progresses, a woman may experience vasomotor symptoms which continue into postmenopausal period.

- According to the **North American Menopause Society**, up to 75% of women in the United States experience hot flashes around menopause. Hot flashes usually occur over a period lasting from 6 months to 2 years but a woman can experience them for up to 10 years.

- The **Study of Women's Health Across the Nations (SWAN) USA** is one of the largest studies to show that prevalence of VMS varies across different ethnic groups with a follow-up of more than 10 yrs.

- In **SWAN** study the highest rate of VMS is seen in African Americans (46%) followed by Hispanics (34%), Whites (31%), Chinese (21%) and Japanese (18%). One important finding from SWAN and other large observational studies is that obesity may be a risk factor rather than a protective characteristic for VMS during perimenopause and early postmenopause.

(B) Mechanism of hot flashes:

Hot flashes are the primary vasomotor symptoms. During flash a sudden sensation of heat affects the upper part of the body e.g. chest, neck and face. The skin in these areas may become red.

Along with hot flashes a woman may experience night sweats, sleep disturbances, anxiety and palpitations. These hot flashes may last for a few seconds to several minutes with average flash lasting about 3 - 6 minutes. Skin temperature may actually rise 1 - 3°F during flash and the core temperature falls slightly.

The sensation is due to rapid dilatation of skin blood vessels which is associated with an increase in metabolic rate and heart rate (↑ 7-15 beats/min) and a reduction in skin resistance. Heart rate and skin blood flow peak within approximately 3 minutes of an onset of a hot flash, which lead to vasodilation and decrease in internal temperature leading to a feel of chill.

No significant changes in blood pressure are associated with hot flashes.

Exact mechanism of VMS is not well understood. Experts believe that following chain of events take place during the phase:

- **Hypothalamic Dysfunction**
  - The hypothalamus contains the thermoregulatory center, which maintains the body's temperature within a narrow range, known as the "thermoregulatory set point."

  - Estrogen deficiency narrows this thermoregulatory zone, making the body more sensitive to slight temperature changes.

  - When the hypothalamus perceives a rise in core temperature—even within the normal range—it triggers mechanisms to dissipate heat, leading to a hot flush.

- **Activation of the Autonomic Nervous System**
  - The hypothalamus activates the autonomic nervous system in response to perceived temperature changes. This activation leads to:
    - ✓ **Vasodilation of skin blood vessels:** This causes an increased blood flow to the skin, producing the characteristic sensation of warmth or heat.

    - ✓ **Sweating:** The body tries to cool itself through evaporative heat loss.

- **Role of Neurotransmitters**
  - Several neurotransmitters, such as **norepinephrine** and **serotonin**, play a role in hot flushes.

  - Changes in norepinephrine levels in the hypothalamus increase the sensitivity of the thermoregulatory center.

  - Serotonin pathways also contribute, influencing the body's response to temperature regulation.

In summary, the mechanism of hot flushes is primarily driven by estrogen deficiency leading to hypothalamic dysfunction and altered thermoregulation. This results in a hypersensitive thermoregulatory center that overreacts to minor temperature fluctuations, causing vasodilation and sweating. Understanding this mechanism is crucial for managing and treating hot flushes effectively.

Grading of hot flashes:

According to the severity, hot flashes are categorised into 3 grades.

- **Mild:** Feeling of heat without sweating
- **Moderate**: Feeling of heat with sweating
- **Severe**: Feeling of heat with sweating and palpitations which disrupts day-to-day usual activities.

VMS as marker:

Frequent and persistent severe VMS have been associated with unfavourable risk factors in relation to health later in life and are surrogate markers of:

- Cardiovascular disease
- Dementia
- Low peak bone mass with subsequent osteoporosis
- All-cause mortality.

Differential Diagnosis of VMS:

- **Medications:**
  - Calcium Channel Blockers
  - Diltiazem
  - Niacin
  - Clomiphene Citrate

- Monosodium Glutamate
- Nitro-glycerine
- Calcitonin
- Raloxifene

- **Diseases:**
  - Thyrotoxicosis
  - Carcinoid syndrome
  - Pheochromocytoma
  - Systemic Mastocytosis
  - Renal Cell Carcinoma
  - Horner's Syndrome

Women should see their health care provider if:

- Hot flashes are moderate to severe and interfere with day- to-day activities.

- They have other symptoms such as diarrhoea, fatigue, unexplained weight loss or general feeling of being unwell.

- They are simultaneously suffering from diabetes or thyroid problems. Health care providers can help women to get treatment to improve their comfort levels and reduce anxiety. Also, they can identify other underlying causes of VMS, if any.

Mild VMS usually do not require any treatment, only counselling and healthy lifestyle modifications can do.

(B) Managing Vasomotor Symptoms (VMS)

As such VMS have a significant impact on the quality of life and overall physical health of women experiencing VMS. Management of vasomotor symptoms include:

- Menopause Hormonal Therapy
- Tibolone
- Nonhormonal Therapy
- Fezolinetant: A New Non-Hormonal Option for Menopausal Symptoms Under Trial
- Complementary Alternative therapy
- Lifestyle changes

Menopause Hormonal Therapy:

- Systemic estrogen therapy remains the most effective treatment for vasomotor symptoms according to the **"2022 Hormone Therapy Position Statement" released by the North American Menopause Society (NAMS).**

- Systemic estrogen with or without progesterone depending upon the presence or absence of uterus should be given in the lowest possible dose and for the shortest possible period to decrease the risk of various adverse long-term events such as thromboembolic disease and breast cancer.

- Most women tolerate MHT, however standard doses are associated with adverse effects like breast tenderness, bloating, headaches, vaginal bleeding etc. Low and ultra-low dose estrogen may improve vasomotor symptoms in some women and have a better adverse effect profile compared with standard doses. There have been limited studies comparing the efficacy of different dosing regimens and hence the treatment should be individualized.

"Initiation of MHT is a safe option for healthy symptomatic women who are within 10 years of menopause or younger than 60 years of age and who do not have other contraindications to MHT." Selection of Estrogen/Progesterone, their dosages, available regimens, duration of therapy everything have been explained thoroughly in previous chapters.

Other Available Options for Vasomotor Symptoms:

1. Tibolone:

Key points:

Tibolone is a unique molecule that exerts weak estrogenic, progestogenic and androgenic properties.

The activity of tibolone and its metabolites is selective and tissue specific and therefore known as **"Selective Tissue Estrogenic Activity Regulator (STEAR)".**

Tibolone itself has no biological activity. Its effects are mediated through its 3 active metabolites.

1. **3 alpha-OH Tibolone -**
2. **3 beta- OH Tibolone -**

Both have affinity for estrogen receptors. Have selective favourable estrogenic effect on bone, vagina but not on breast and endometrium.

3. delta- 4- Isomer -

Shows affinity for both progesterone and androgen receptors, showing progestogenic effect on endometrium and androgenic effect for improving libido and sexual function.

Tibolone-Structure And Mechanism Of Action

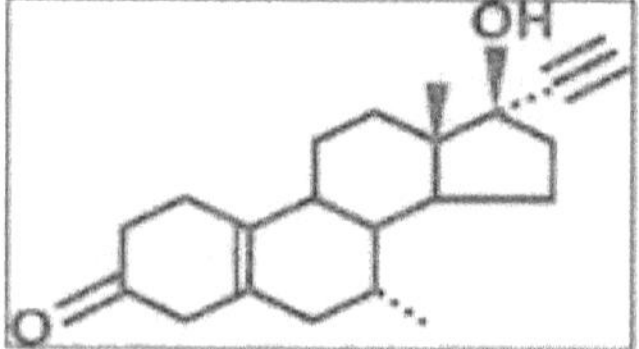

Tibolone is a selective tissue oestrogenic activity regulator

Kinetics

Metabolism of Tibolone

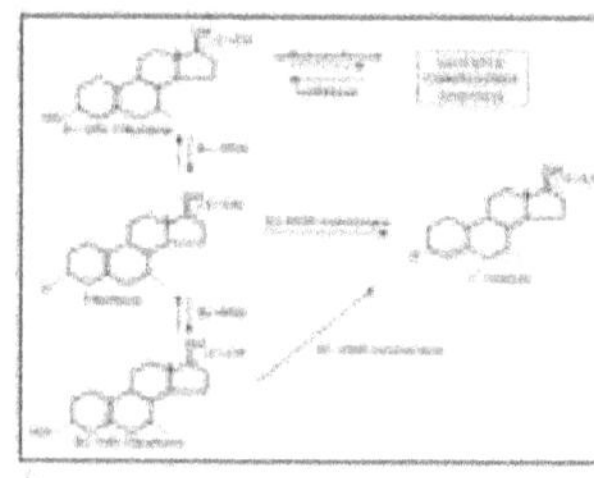

- Rapid and extensive absorption
- Rapid metabolism to
  - 3α-OH-tibolone
  - 3β-OH-tibolone
  - Δ4-isomer of tibolone
- Excretion is mainly as conjugated (sulfated) metabolites
- Kinetics are not affected by food or renal function

Tissue-Specific Effects Of Tibolone's Metabolites

Specific binding affinities of tibolone and its primary metabolites

Tibolone/ Metabolites	Oestrogen Receptor	Progestogen Receptor	Androgen Receptor
Tibolone	+	+	+
3-alpha-hydroxy tibolone/ 3-beta-hydroxy tibolone	+	-	-
Δ^4 Tibolone	-	+	+

+ Stimulatory effect; - Suppressive effect; ? Unknown effect

Tibolone is approved in 90 countries to treat menopausal symptoms.

Tibolone has been used for almost 20 years in Europe for the treatment of vasomotor symptoms but it is not available in the United States.

A double blind randomised controlled trial of 437 postmenopausal women found that treatment with tibolone significantly reduced the mean score for hot flashes and was comparable with estrogen therapy.

Tibolone increases the risk of recurrence of breast cancer in a woman with breast cancer survivors.

It may increase the risk of stroke in a woman over 60 years of age.

Pharmacokinetics of tibolone:

- Tibolone is rapidly and almost completely absorbed orally, plasma levels are detectable within 30 minutes and peak levels reach within 1 to 1.5 hrs.

- Majority of tibolone (96.3%) is protein bound and it has considerably lower affinity (<2.5%) for SHBG than testosterone.

- Mainly excreted via faeces (60-65%).

- Drug interactions: It enhances warfarin-induced anticoagulant effects and therefore simultaneous use of tibolone and warfarin should be monitored and warfarin dose adjusted if necessary.

- High fat meal reduces tibolone absorption and metabolite formation.

Beneficial Effects of Tibolone:

- Relieves climacteric symptoms.
  Effectively controls hot flashes, night sweats, fatigue, nervousness, headache and insomnia.

- Positively affects mood and improves sexual well-being.

- Induces a healthy vaginal environment.

- Improves vaginal cytology and cervical mucus production.

- Reduces vaginal dryness and dyspareunia.

- Prevents bone loss and increases BMD even in women with established osteoporosis.

Safety profile of tibolone:

Tibolone does not stimulate endometrium.

- **THEBES study (Tibolone Histology of Endometrium and Breast Endpoint Study)** was a prospective, randomised clinical trial designed to provide the endometrial safety of tibolone compared with EPT. Endometrial histology shows a low prevalence of endometrial hyperplasia (0.18%) and no carcinomas.

- A delta-4- isomer of tibolone exerts progestogenic action on the endometrium.

- By inhibiting 17 beta-HSD (type 1) and sulfatase, levels of local estrogens are reduced and estrones are also converted into inactive estrogens respectively.

- Combination of reduced levels of estrogen and the strong progestogenic action ensures no endometrial stimulation.

Tibolone does not increase the mammographic density of the breast:

- Inhibitory effect on enzyme sulfatase is tissue selective and is strong in the human breast cell lines (70-90%), weaker in human endometrial cell lines (8 - 43%) and absent in human osteoblast-like cell lines.

- Tibolone and its metabolites also reduce proliferation and increase apoptosis in normal human breast epithelial cells.

- There is a low incidence of vaginal bleeding compared to the E+P MHT regimen - a need of every woman.

- Proven 10 years safety.

Tibolone as add-back therapy in women on GnRH agonists:

- GnRH agonists are used in endometriosis and myomas in premenopausal women. This can cause severe suppression of estrogens leading to temporary **'Estrogen Deficiency Syndrome'.** Patients may experience symptoms like hot flushes, bone loss etc., forcing them to stop GnRH agonist therapy. In such cases if tibolone is used as add-back therapy, it can cause symptomatic relief without adverse effects.

Tibolone dosage:

- Single daily dose is 2.5 mg, taken preferably at the same time. 1.25 mg has also been found equally effective.

- **In natural menopause it is to be started at least 12 months postmenopause.** If started in perimenopause, it can give rise to irregular bleeding with menorrhagia. In surgical menopause it can be started immediately.

- If you want to switch from MHT to Tibolone, then in case of sequential MHT regimen, start tibolone on the day following completion of prior regimen while in case of continuous combined regimen start tibolone at any time.

- In case of a missed dose, take it as soon as you remember.
  If > 12 hrs overdue, skip dose, next dose at normal time.
  Missing dose may increase chances of breakthrough bleeding/spotting.

Side Effects:

- Nausea, but usually mild and self-limiting.

- Sometimes breakthrough bleeding/spotting may occur. It is not necessary to investigate if bleeding occurs within 3 months of treatment unless severe.

- Transitory breast tenderness may occur,

- Weight gain

- It causes reduction in HDL-C levels.

Contraindications:

- Known, past or suspected breast cancer.
- Known or suspected estrogen-dependent cancers.
- Undiagnosed genital bleeding.
- Thromboembolic disease
- Severe liver disease
- Pregnancy

In conclusion, apart from relief from vasomotor symptoms tibolone may have added value in women with:

- Risk of accelerated bone loss
- Urogenital complaints
- Low sex drive
- Premenopausal breast tenderness
- Mammographically high breast density
- Mood disorders
- Fibroids

2. Nonhormonal therapy for vasomotor symptoms:

- Estrogen is the most effective treatment available to relieve bothersome symptoms of menopause.

- However, nonhormonal management of VMS is an important consideration when hormone therapy is not an option either because of medical contraindications or a woman's personal choice.

- ***The 2015 NICE guidelines made it very clear that SSRI or SNRI should not be used as first-line treatment of severe VMS in women who have no contraindications for MHT.***

- Clinicians need to know currently available nonhormonal management options of VMS.

- Although non-estrogen treatment may not be as effective as estrogen therapy, they do provide considerable relief.

Following non- hormonal medications are available.

Antidepressants:

- **SSRI** (Selective Serotonin Receptor Inhibitors)
- **SNRI** (Serotonin and Norepinephrine Reuptake Inhibitors)

Anticonvulsants:

- Gabapentin
- Pregabalin

Antihypertensive agent:

- Clonidine

Anticholinergic agent:

- Oxybutynin

Antidepressants:

Antidepressant medications are recommended as a first line treatment for hot flashes in women for whom estrogen is contraindicated or who are not willing for MHT because of the fear of its side effects.

SSRI (Selective Serotonin Receptor Inhibitors):

SSRIs are the class of antidepressants used most commonly for treating hot flashes.

Paroxetine:

- Paroxetine is the only nonhormonal therapy that is specifically approved for hot flashes by USFDA. This medication has been used for many years for treating depression, but can be effective in lower doses for hot flashes.
- A recent 2015 published RCT conducted over a period of 1 year treated for VMS showed that paroxetine 7.5 mg/day significantly reduces the number of night awakenings attributed to VMS.
- Women with breast cancer who are taking tamoxifen, should not take paroxetine as it can interfere with tamoxifen action, thus reducing its efficacy.

Fluoxetine:

- A double blind randomised cross over study showed a 50% decrease in hot flashes in fluoxetine group versus 30% reduction in placebo group. The recommended dose is 10 - 30 mg/day.

Citalopram:

- Tested for hot flashes in a pilot trial in 2003 which involved 26 women with the history of breast cancer. In a 4 weeks treatment schedule 10 mg daily for the first week and 20 mg daily for the following weeks, the patient had a decrease in hot flashes frequency by 58%.

SNRI (Serotonin and Norepinephrine Reuptake Inhibitors):

Venlafaxine and Desvenlafaxine:

- Are known to improve mood, and may also impact thermoregulation.
- The optimum results have been with Venlafaxine 75 mg SR and Desvenlafaxine 100 mg.
- 75 mg Venlafaxine is equivalent to an ultra-low dose of estrogen (25 mcg) for the treatment of hot flashes.
- Venlafaxine should not be used in women with heart disease, electrolyte imbalance and uncontrolled high blood pressure.

American Cancer Society (ACS) and the American Society of Clinical Oncology (ASCO) recommend that primary care clinicians should offer SSRI and SNRI for hot flashes relief in breast cancer survivors.

Adverse effects with SSRIs and SNRIs, which usually go away with time or with a change in doses; include nausea, dizziness, dry mouth, nervousness, constipation, somnolence and sexual dysfunction. SNRIs may have slightly more side effects than SSRIs.

Anticonvulsants:

- **Gabapentin:**
  Gabapentin is a medication that has been developed to treat seizures. It also relieves hot flashes in some women. The recommended daily dose for hot flashes is

300 mg thrice daily or 900 mg at bedtime. This reduces symptoms by 45%. Side effects include dizziness and peripheral oedema.

- **Pregabalin:**
  Pregabalin is a new generation compound with a mechanism of action similar to Gabapentin. The recommended dose is 75 mg at bedtime, and can increase to 150 mg twice daily. Adverse effects include dizziness, drowsiness, nausea, and headache.

Antihypertensive agent:

- **Clonidine:**
  Clonidine basically is a centrally acting antihypertensive drug. It has been found to reduce hot flashes by 15-20% compared with placebo in women with a history of breast cancer. To start with, the dose 25 mcg twice daily, can be increased to 50-75 mcg twice daily.

Anticholinergic agent:

- **Oxybutynin:**
  Oxybutynin is used to treat overactive bladder and urinary incontinence. It has been demonstrated to be effective in treating hot flashes and night sweats. Usually started with a 5 mg tablet at bedtime, can be increased slowly to 5 mg twice daily for at least 5 weeks. The most bothersome side effects are dry mouth, dry eyes, blurred vision, dizziness and drowsiness.

3. Fezolinetant: A New Non-Hormonal Option for Menopausal Symptoms

Fezolinetant is an emerging non-hormonal therapy designed to address menopausal symptoms, particularly vasomotor symptoms (VMS), such as hot flashes and night sweats. These symptoms are common during menopause due to fluctuating and declining estrogen levels, impacting quality of life for many women. Unlike traditional hormone replacement therapy (HRT), Fezolinetant offers a novel mechanism of action that avoids hormonal pathways, making it an appealing option for women who cannot or prefer not to use HRT.

Mechanism of Action

Fezolinetant is a selective neurokinin-3 (NK3) receptor antagonist. Neurokinin B, a neuropeptide, plays a key role in the thermoregulatory center of the hypothalamus, where it contributes to the dysregulation seen in menopausal VMS. By blocking NK3 receptors, Fezolinetant helps restore balance in the hypothalamic thermoregulatory pathways, reducing the frequency and severity of hot flashes and night sweats.

Key Benefits

- **Non-Hormonal:** Suitable for women who cannot use estrogen-based therapies, such as those with a history of hormone-sensitive cancers, thromboembolic disorders, or other contraindications to HRT.

- **Targeted Action:** Specifically addresses VMS without systemic hormonal effects.

- **Potential for Broad Use:** Expands treatment options for women who prefer alternative therapies or do not tolerate HRT.

Clinical Efficacy

- Clinical trials have demonstrated significant reductions in the frequency and severity of hot flashes in women treated with Fezolinetant compared to placebo.

- Improvements were often observed within the first few weeks of treatment, with sustained benefits over time.

Safety Profile

- Fezolinetant has been well-tolerated in clinical studies, with common side effects being mild and including headache, nausea, and fatigue.

- As a non-hormonal option, it does not carry the risks associated with estrogen therapy, such as increased risks of breast cancer, thromboembolism, or endometrial hyperplasia.

Potential Implications

- The introduction of Fezolinetant marks a significant advancement in the management of menopausal symptoms. It provides a safe and effective alternative for women who:
    - Have contraindications to HRT.
    - Prefer non-hormonal treatments.
    - Are looking for rapid symptom relief without systemic hormonal exposure.

In summary, Fezolinetant represents a promising option in the evolving landscape of menopause management. Its non-hormonal approach, combined with efficacy in reducing VMS, makes it a valuable tool for improving the quality of life in menopausal women. As more long-term data become available, Fezolinetant is likely to further solidify its role as a cornerstone therapy for menopausal symptoms.

4. Complementary Alternative Therapy:

Phytoestrogens

Phytoestrogens are plant-derived compounds that mimic estrogen in the body. They are found in foods and supplements and can alleviate vasomotor symptoms.

- **Sources:**
  - **Soy Isoflavones:** Found in soybeans, tofu, and soy milk.
  - **Flaxseed (Lignans):** Ground flaxseed can be added to meals.
  - **Red Clover:** Contains isoflavones; available as teas or supplements.
- **Effectiveness:**
  - Mixed results from studies, but some show moderate reduction in hot flashes and night sweats.
  - Generally safe when consumed in dietary amounts.
- **Considerations:**
  - Effectiveness depends on the individual's ability to metabolize phytoestrogens.
  - Use with caution in women with hormone-sensitive cancers.

Herbal Treatments

Herbal remedies are widely used to manage menopausal symptoms, including vasomotor symptoms.

- **Common Herbs:**
    - **Black Cohosh (Cimicifuga racemosa):** Popular for reducing hot flashes and night sweats.
    - **Evening Primrose Oil:** May help with night sweats but lacks consistent evidence.
    - **Dong Quai:** Traditional Chinese herb, though evidence is inconclusive.
    - **Ginseng:** Can improve mood and sleep quality but has limited effects on hot flashes.
    - **Maca Root:** May help balance hormones and reduce symptoms.
    - **Chaste Tree Berry (Vitex agnus-castus):** Regulates hormonal imbalances.

- **Precautions:**
    - Quality and purity of herbal products can vary.
    - Possible interactions with medications; consult a healthcare provider.

Acupuncture:

- Studies show acupuncture can reduce the frequency and severity of hot flashes.
- May also improve sleep quality and overall well-being.

Hypnotherapy:

- Can reduce hot flash intensity and frequency.
- Involves guided relaxation and suggestion techniques.

Cognitive Behavioral Therapy (CBT):

- Effective in managing the emotional impact of vasomotor symptoms.
- Helps in reframing thoughts around symptoms and improving coping mechanisms.

Homeopathy:

- Remedies such as Sepia, Lachesis, or Sulphur are often recommended, but scientific evidence is limited.

In summary, while alternative and complementary treatments can help alleviate vasomotor symptoms, their effectiveness varies among individuals. It's essential to consult with a healthcare provider, especially if combining these therapies with conventional hormone therapy, to ensure safety and avoid potential interactions.

Lifestyle modifications to get relief from hot flashes:

Lifestyle modifications can play a significant role in reducing the severity and frequency of vasomotor symptoms (hot flashes and night sweats) experienced during menopause. Here's a comprehensive guide:

1. Maintain a Healthy Diet

A balanced diet can help stabilize hormones and reduce triggers for vasomotor symptoms.

- **Increase Intake of:**
  - **Fruits and Vegetables:** Rich in antioxidants and phytonutrients.
  - **Whole Grains:** Provide steady energy and prevent blood sugar spikes.
  - **Omega-3 Fatty Acids:** Found in fatty fish, flaxseed, and walnuts, they may reduce inflammation and improve mood.
  - **Phytoestrogens:** Include soy products (tofu, soy milk), flaxseeds, and chickpeas to help mimic estrogen effects.

- **Limit or Avoid:**

  - **Caffeine and Alcohol:** Known triggers for hot flashes.
  - **Spicy Foods:** Can exacerbate symptoms in some women.
  - **Sugary and Processed Foods:** Can cause blood sugar fluctuations, worsening symptoms.
  - **Smoking** increases the risk of severe vasomotor symptoms and contributes to other health issues like heart disease and osteoporosis. Quitting smoking can significantly improve symptoms.

2. Stay Hydrated

- **Water Intake:** Aim for at least 8-10 glasses of water daily to help regulate body temperature and replace fluids lost during night sweats.

3. Dress Strategically

- **Lightweight, Breathable Fabrics:**
  - Opt for cotton, linen, or moisture-wicking fabrics.
  - Avoid synthetic materials that trap heat.

- **Layering:**
  - Wear layers that can be easily removed during a hot flash.

- **Nightwear and Bedding:**
  - Use lightweight pajamas and breathable sheets.
  - Consider cooling pillows and a fan near your bed.

4. Optimize Your Sleep Environment

- **Bedroom Temperature:**
  - Keep the room cool (around 60–67°F or 16–19°C).
  - Use fans or air conditioning as needed.

- **Relaxation Before Bed:**
  - Establish a calming bedtime routine to reduce stress.
  - Avoid screens and heavy meals 2–3 hours before bed.

5. Manage Stress

Stress can trigger or worsen hot flashes. Adopting stress-reduction techniques can help:

- **Mindfulness and Meditation:**
  - Practice deep breathing exercises or guided meditation to calm the mind.

- **Yoga or Tai Chi:**
  - Helps reduce stress and improve mood while enhancing flexibility and balance.

6. Regular Exercise

Exercise improves overall health and can help manage vasomotor symptoms.

- **Aerobic Exercise:**
  - Walking, jogging, swimming, or cycling enhances circulation and regulates body temperature.

- **Strength Training:**
  - Helps maintain bone density and muscle mass post-menopause.

- **Stretching and Relaxation:**
  - Yoga or Pilates can promote relaxation and improve sleep quality.

7. Practice Relaxation Techniques

Relaxation techniques can help manage stress and reduce the intensity of symptoms.

- **Deep Breathing:**
  - Engage in slow, deep breaths at the onset of a hot flash.
  - A pattern of inhaling for 4 seconds, holding for 7 seconds, and exhaling for 8 seconds can be helpful.

- **Progressive Muscle Relaxation:**
  - Sequentially tensing and relaxing muscle groups helps reduce tension.

8. Maintain a Healthy Weight

- Being overweight can worsen vasomotor symptoms. Losing weight through a healthy diet and exercise may help alleviate hot flashes and improve overall well-being.

9. Regular Medical Check-ups

- Regular visits to your healthcare provider ensure that other underlying health issues, such as thyroid disorders or anxiety, are ruled out or managed.

10. Social Support

- Share your experiences with friends, family, or a support group.
- Talking about symptoms and coping strategies can reduce stress and feelings of isolation.

These lifestyle modifications, along with a positive mindset, can significantly improve the quality of life during menopause and reduce the impact of vasomotor symptoms.

CHAPTER VI: MANAGEMENT OF UROGENITAL SYMPTOMS OF MENOPAUSE (GSM)

Taking care of your body

is a form of self-respect.

– Anonymous

(A) Definition of GSM

Genitourinary system of menopause is defined as a collection of signs and symptoms associated with decrease in estrogen and other sex steroids leading to changes in labia majora, labia minora, clitoris, vagina, urethra, bladder, introitus and vestibule.

Symptoms of GSM:

- **Genital Symptoms (70 %)**
    - Vaginal dryness
    - Itching
    - Burning and irritation
    - Vaginal spotting
    - Discharge
    - Vaginal vault prolapses
    - Cracks over perineum

- **Urinary Symptoms (40 – 60 %)**
    - Urgency
    - Frequency
    - Urinary incontinency
    - Dysuria
    - Nocturia
    - RUTs (Recurrent Urinary Tract Infections)

- **Sexual Symptoms (35 – 60 %)**
    - Lack of lubrication
    - Dyspareunia
    - Decreased arousal
    - Loss of libido
    - Orgasm difficulties

Important Facts about GSM

- The genitourinary system of menopause (GSM) is a relatively new terminology for the conditions previously described as:
    - **Vulvovaginal Atrophy**
    - **Atrophic Vaginitis**
    - **Urogenital Atrophy**

- The new terminology GSM was first introduced in 2014 by a consensus of the **International Society for the Study of Women's Sexual Health (ISSWSH)** and the **North American Society.**

- GSM is the correct terminology as it describes the spectrum of changes in the genitourinary system as a whole due to the deficiency of endogenous estrogen in menopause.

- Prevalence of GSM or its features manifest in approximately:
    - 15 % of perimenopausal women
    - 40 – 54 % of postmenopausal women

- GSM is a chronic progressive condition and typically does not resolve of its own unless treated in time.

- Symptoms are not life-threatening, but they are progressive and have a profound impact on the quality of life of postmenopausal women by negatively affecting self-esteem and intimacy with their partners.

- GSM is inevitable as it is an aging process but treatment in time is of paramount importance for preventing the exacerbations of the symptoms.

- GSM still remains an underdiagnosed and consequently undertreated condition despite its high prevalence as most of the menopausal women do not seek help at the very onset of symptoms. This may be because of:

    - The reluctance among women to seek help due to embarrassment,

      Or

    - The result of the tendency among many women to consider it as a normal feature of aging process,

      Or

    - Unaware of the fact that the condition can get relief with the available medications.

Symptoms of GSM affect the quality of life of a postmenopausal woman. Symptoms differ from woman to woman. Not all above-described symptoms are seen in all women.

(B) Normal health of vagina and lower urinary tract:

- The female genital tract and lower urinary tract arise from common embryological origin – **Urogenital Sinus**. Both are sensitive to the effects of sex steroid hormones and share common susceptibility to estrogen deprivation.

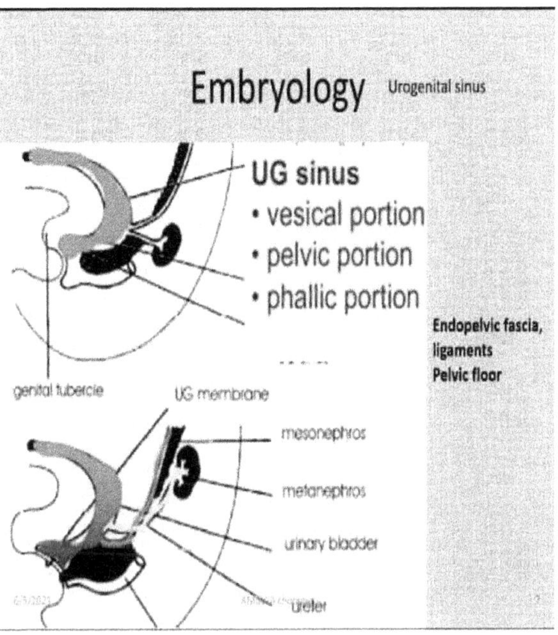

- Density of estrogen receptors is highest in vagina while it is less across external genitalia to the skin.

- Density of androgen receptors is reverse. They are at low levels in vagina and higher levels across external genitalia.

- Progesterone receptors are found in vagina and transitional epithelium of the vulvovaginal junction.

- Vaginal cytology is quantified by **"Vaginal Maturation Index" (VMI),** a ratio of superficial, intermediate and parabasal cells from the upper one third of vagina.

- Estrogen helps to sustain the thickness of the multi-layered squamous epithelium which imparts normal pink colour, rugae and moisture.

- Estrogen promotes glycogen formation in superficial cells of squamous epithelium.

- Doderlein Lactobacilli are a part of normal vaginal flora and convert this glycogen into lactic acid, thus keeping vaginal pH < 4.5 in postmenopausal women. This acidic pH serves to reduce the vaginal infection.

- Normal healthy vaginal secretions come from:
    - Fluid transudation from blood vessels.
    - Secretion from cervical glands and
    - Secretion from Bartholin's gland.

(C) Pathophysiology of GSM:

- Estradiol level in the menopausal women is < 20 pg /ml, while in premenopausal women it ranges from 40 – 400 pg/ml depending upon the stage of the cycle.

- Vaginal tissues of the postmenopausal women have enzymes:
    - 17 Beta HSD (hydroxysteroid dehydrogenase) Type 2 that oxidises estradiol to less active estrone.

    - Estrone sulfotransferase converts estradiol to inactive estrone sulphate.

    - Vagina is the most accessible and surrogate indicator of low estrogen levels.

    - Like estrogen, serum androgen and DHEA markedly decrease with age and so in menopausal women. Approximately 60 % of androgen present at 30 years of age is lost at the time of menopause, with serum DHEA showing similar decline.

- Due to estrogen deficiency and breakdown of collagen support, thinning of vaginal epithelium becomes apparent 2 – 3 years after menopause. There is decreased blood flow to the tissues.

- As atrophic changes start developing, there is decrease in exfoliated glycogen containing superficial cells with concurrent increase in proportion of para basal cells.

- Due to decrease availability of glycogen from superficial cells and also changes in vaginal flora (decrease in Doderlein lactobacilli); enough lactic acid is not produced to maintain acidic ph.

- Finally vaginal pH increases to over 6, thus exposing postmenopausal vagina at increased risk of infection, increased vulnerability to physical irritation and trauma.

- Urethral mucosa atrophies and the collagen content in the connective tissue surrounding the urethra also decreases. Blood flow in urethra is also reduced. All these changes including changes in vaginal flora predispose postmenopausal women to recurrent urinary tract infections (RUTIs) by a variety of pathogens.

Pathophysiology of GSM:

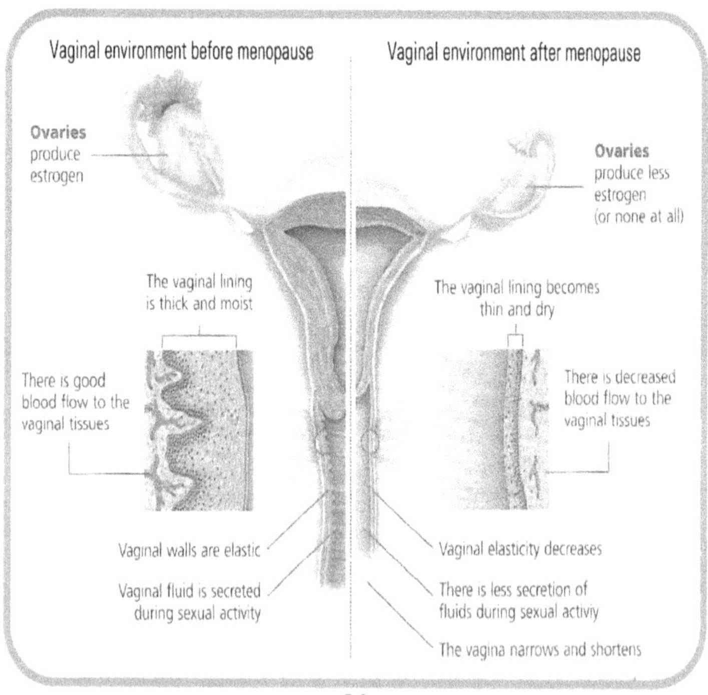

Reference :
Johnston L. The Recognition and Management of Atrophic Vaginitis. *Geriatrics & Aging* 2002; 5(7):9-15.

- **Vulva**
  - Becomes flattened and thin due to loss of collagen and adipose tissue.
  - Epithelial glands are attenuated, diminished secretions from sebaceous glands.
  - Clitoris atrophies.
  - Clitoris glans loses protective covering and is irritated more easily with any type of contact (e.g. clothing, prolong sitting, sexual contact).
- **Vagina**
  - Thinner, less elastic, pale, progressively smoother with loss of rugae.
  - Fewer secretions, delayed onset of lubrication during sexual stimulation.
- **Vaginal surface**
  - Friable.
  - Petechial, ulcerations and bleeding after minimal trauma.
  - Healing adhesions may develop between touching surfaces.
- **Vaginal epithelium**
  - Decreased ratio of superficial cells to para basal cells.
  - Decreased blood flow.

- **Vaginal canal**
    - Shorter, narrower.

- **Urethra**
    - Urethral meatal prominence

    - Thinning of urethral epithelium

- **Vaginal ph**
    - **> 5**

Source: *Bachmann GA, et. al. Treatment of postmenopausal women: Basic and Clinical Aspects, 1999.195-201. Semmens JP et. al. Obstet Gynecol, 1985; 66: 15-18.*

Risk Factors for GSM:

- **Deficiency of oestrogen causes GSM. Low estrogen states in women's life include:**
    - Natural menopause
    - Surgical menopause
    - Premature ovarian failure
    - Postpartum period (breast feeding)
    - Hypothalamic amenorrhoea
    - Medicines having antiestrogenic effect include:
        - Tamoxifen
        - Danazol
        - GnRh agonist

- **Cancer treatment including pelvic irradiation, chemotherapy.**

- **Exacerbating factors for GSM**
    - Vaginal nulliparity
    - Sexual abstinence

- Cigarette smoking
- Alcohol abuse
- Previous vaginal surgery
- Feminine hygiene spray, deodorants.

(D) Diagnosis of GSM:

GSM is a clinical diagnosis based on a constellation of genital, sexual and urinary symptoms and examination findings. No further testing or work-up is necessary.

- **History and examination**

  - Symptoms and their severity.

  - Per speculum examination with small size speculum
    - External genitalia
    - Vagina
    - Cervix

  - Gentle one finger examination to palpate cervix and uterus.

  - Signs: Look for all anatomical changes due to atrophy as described above. The classic appearance of vaginal atrophy includes loss of rugae and a pale thin vaginal epithelium, tenderness on palpation, reduced vaginal elasticity, narrowing and shortening of vagina and an increased susceptibility to trauma.

  - Wet-mount microscopy: Immature vaginal epithelial cells with large nuclei (para basal cells), minimal or absent lactobacilli and > 1 WBC per epithelial cell.

  - Vaginal ph testing: Place a paper indicator strip in vagina to test whether ph is > 5.

- Modified Vaginal Health Index: Minimum the total score, severe is the atrophy.

- PAP smear to rule out Ca-Cx.

- TVS to measure ET and to rule out other uterine pathology, if any.

- Urine routine and C/S, if having urinary symptoms.

- **Modified Vaginal Health Index:**

  - Modified vaginal index assesses 7 parameters.
  - Parameters are graded from 1 to 3, and total score ranges from 7 to 21.
  - The minimum total score of 7 points includes severe vulvovaginal atrophy.
  - Parameters and scoring are illustrated in the following table.

Modified Vaginal Health Index

Parameters	**1**	**2**	**3**
Ph	>6.5	5-6.5	<5
Moisture	No	Minimal	Good
Rugosity	None	Minimal	Good
Elasticity	Poor	Fair	Excellent
Length of vagina	<4cms	4-6 cms	>6 cms
Epithelial integrity	Petechae	Petechae after scraping	Normal
Vascularity	Minimal	Fair	Good

(E) Management of GSM:

- **Goal for management:**
    - Relief of symptoms
    - Restoration of vaginal physiology

- **Management options:**

    1. **Lifestyle modifications**
    2. **Nonhormone therapy**
        - Vaginal lubricants
        - Vaginal moisturizers
    3. **Hormone therapy**
        - Local vaginal estrogen therapy **(Gold Standard)**
    4. **Others include:**
        - Tibolone
        - Ospemifene
        - Dehydroepiandrosterone Acetate (DHEA)
        - Phytoestrogen
        - Laser therapy

Lifestyle Modifications:

Adopting healthy habits can help maintain the integrity and function of the genitourinary system and alleviate GSM symptoms.

- **Personal Hygiene:**
    - Use gentle, unscented soaps or pH-balanced washes specifically designed for intimate areas.

    - Avoid douching, as it disrupts the natural vaginal microbiota.

- Wear breathable, cotton-based underwear and avoid tight-fitting clothes.

- **Diet and Hydration:**
  - Stay hydrated to support tissue hydration and urinary health.
  - Incorporate foods rich in **phytoestrogens** (e.g., soy, flaxseeds) to mimic estrogen-like activity.
  - Consume a balanced diet with adequate **omega-3 fatty acids** (e.g., fish, nuts) for anti-inflammatory benefits.

- **Sexual Activity:**
  - Sexual activity is the healthy prescription for postmenopausal women. Continued vaginal coitus provides protection from urogenital atrophy, presumably by increasing the blood flow to the pelvic organs.
  - Masturbation also increases genital blood flow in menopausal women and may benefit to sustain urogenital health.
  - Regular sexual activity, with or without a partner, helps maintain vaginal elasticity and blood flow.
  - Use of appropriate lubricants during intercourse to reduce friction and pain.

- **Physical Activity:**
  - Engage in regular pelvic floor exercises (e.g., Kegels) to strengthen the pelvic muscles and improve urinary control.
  - Maintain a healthy weight to reduce pressure on the pelvic region.

- **Smoking Cessation:**
  Since GSM is the end result of estrogen deficiency, lifestyle factors that hasten this decline may be avoided. As smoking fastens the oestrogen metabolism and is associated with reduced blood flow and higher rates of vaginal atrophy, smoking cessation would delay / prevent vaginal atrophy.

- Regular drinking of cranberry juice may reduce the risk of recurrence of UTI.

- Vaginal dilators may improve vaginal function for those who have desire for vaginal intercourse but in whom estrogen therapy is contraindicated.

Nonhormone Therapy:

Vaginal Lubricants and the moisturizers are the first-line treatments for GSM, especially for those unable or unwilling to use hormone therapy.

Vaginal Lubricants:

- **Purpose:**
  - Provide temporary relief from dyspareunia and dryness during sexual activity.

- **Characteristics:**
  - Water-based, silicone-based, or oil-based options are available.

  - Non-irritating and free from fragrances or additives.

- **Common Products:**
  - **Water-based lubricants**: Easy to clean but may require reapplication (e.g., KY Jelly).

- **Silicone-based lubricants**: Longer-lasting and ideal for severe dryness (e.g., Uber lube).
- **Oil-based lubricants**: Long-lasting but may not be compatible with latex condoms.

- **Usage:**
  - Apply externally and internally before sexual activity.

- **Avoid:**
  - Women who are prone for vaginal fungal infection should avoid glycerine-based lubricants.
  - Avoid petroleum jelly or other petroleum-based products for lubrication if also using condoms, because petroleum can break down latex condoms on contact.

Vaginal Moisturizers:

- **Purpose:**
  - Provide long-term hydration and improve vaginal elasticity by restoring moisture to the vaginal tissues.

- **Characteristics:**
  - Designed for regular use, typically 2–3 times per week, irrespective of sexual activity.
  - Mimics natural vaginal secretions to relieve dryness and discomfort.
  - Have buffering properties which reduce vaginal ph.

- **Common Ingredients:**
    - **Hyaluronic acid**: A hydrating agent that retains moisture.
    - **Polycarbophil-based products**: Adhere to the vaginal wall and provide sustained hydration (e.g., Replens).
- **Usage:**
    - Apply intravaginally using an applicator as per product instructions.

Vaginal lubricants and moisturizers provide temporary relief and may be sufficient for patients with mild symptoms. Contraindicated only in women with an allergic reaction to a particular product.

Key Differences Between Lubricants and Moisturizers

Aspect	Lubricants	Moisturizers
Purpose	Temporary relief during intercourse	Long-term hydration and elasticity
Duration	Short-term, immediate effect	Long-lasting, regular maintenance
Application	Before sexual activity	2–3 times per week regularly

Hormone Therapy (Local vaginal estrogen therapy)

- ***Gold standard** for the treatment of GSM.*
  - Should be started early to prevent irreversible atrophic changes and may need long term treatment to maintain long term benefits.
  - Estrogen is easily absorbed through atrophic vaginal epithelium and causes maturation. As the epithelium matures, absorption decreases, thus smaller doses are then required to maintain vaginal health and restoration of vaginal ph.
  - Local vaginal estrogen does not cause much increase in serum estrogen levels; therefore, no endometrial hyperplasia and no endometrial surveillance is required.
  - No progesterone supplement is required as there is no endometrial hyperplasia.
- Unscheduled vaginal bleeding should be investigated by an ultrasound and endometrial sampling.
- **Mode of Action:**

Local estrogen therapy works by replenishing estrogen levels in the vaginal and lower urinary tract tissues, leading to structural and functional improvements.

- **Effects on Vaginal Epithelium:**
  - Increases epithelial thickness by stimulating cell proliferation.
  - Restores glycogen production in epithelial cells.

- Glycogen serves as a substrate for Lactobacilli, promoting lactic acid production and maintaining an acidic vaginal pH.

- Enhances tissue hydration and lubrication by improving glandular function.

- **Effects on Connective Tissue:**
  - Increases collagen, elastin, and hyaluronic acid levels, improving elasticity, strength, and moisture retention.

- **Effects on Vascularization:**
  - Promotes angiogenesis and improves blood flow to the vaginal tissues, reducing hypoxia and enhancing tissue repair.

- **Effects on Microbiota:**
  - Restores an acidic pH (3.5–4.5) by promoting Lactobacilli dominance, preventing infections like bacterial vaginosis or urinary tract infections.

- **Effects on Lower Urinary Tract:**
  - Improves urethral mucosal thickness and vascularization.

  - Reduces symptoms such as urinary urgency, frequency, incontinence, and recurrent urinary tract infections.

- **Follow-up and duration of treatment:**

  Regular follow-up ensures treatment efficacy and addresses any concerns or potential adverse effects.
  - **Initial Follow-Up:**
    - **Timeline:** 4–6 weeks after starting therapy.

- **Purpose:**
  - ✓ Assess symptom relief (dryness, dyspareunia, urinary symptoms).
  - ✓ Check for local irritation, discharge, or other side effects.
  - ✓ Ensure proper application technique and adherence to treatment.

- **Subsequent Follow-Up:**
  - **Timeline:** Every 6–12 months for maintenance therapy.
  - **Purpose:**
    - ✓ Monitor symptom control and quality of life.
    - ✓ Evaluate vaginal health through physical examination (vaginal pH, epithelial integrity).
    - ✓ Rule out rare side effects such as endometrial stimulation (especially in patients with a uterus).
    - ✓ Reinforce the importance of adherence to the maintenance regimen.

- **Long-Term Monitoring:**
  - Patients on long-term therapy require periodic reassessment to determine the continued need for therapy.
  - Evaluate for any new contraindications or comorbidities.

Commercially available low dose vaginal preparations:

Type	Brand name	Composition	Starting dose	Maintenance
Cream	Evalon	Estriol 1 mg/1 gm	o.5-1 gm daily for 2 weeks	0.5-1 gm twice weekly
Cream	Premarin	CEE 0.625/1 gm	0.5-1 gm daily for 2 weeks	0.5-1 gm twice weekly
Cream	Estrace	17 beta Estradiol 0.1mg/1 gm	0.5-1 gm daily for 2 weeks	0.5-1 gm twice weekly
Tablets/ Inserts	Vegifem Imvexxy	Estradiol hemihydrate 4 mcg, 10 mcg	One tablet daily for 2 weeks	One tablet twice a week
Vaginal Ring	Estring	17 beta Estradiol 2mg impregnated in ring	Releases 7.5 mcg/day	Replace ring after 90 days

- **Safety and Considerations**
    - **Safety Profile:**
        - Minimal systemic absorption, making it safe for most women.
        - Safety data up to 1 year is available.

- Various studies concluded that cream, gel, tablet, inserts and rings all appear to be equally effective in alleviating signs and symptoms of GSM, but differ slightly in effect profile. Applying vaginal cream may feel messy for many women. They may use inserts / tablets. Vaginal rings are well tolerated and do not interfere with sexual intercourse.

- **Adverse Effects:**
  Rare and localized, including mild irritation, spotting, or discharge.

- **Contraindications:**
  Untreated endometrial hyperplasia or estrogen-sensitive cancers (requires individualized assessment).

- **Studies on the safety of the use of vaginal oestrogen in GSM**

  - Two large prospective **US Cohort Study** in postmenopausal women provides reassurance regarding safety of vaginal oestrogen.

  - **WHI (Women Health Initiative Study):**
    Followed over 1500 women who used vaginal estrogen for median duration of 2 years.

  - **Nurse Health Study:**
    900 postmenopausal women who used vaginal oestrogen for median duration of 3 years.

In neither of these studies, women had elevated risk of endometrial, or colorectal cancer. No elevated risk of CHD, Stroke, VTE.

- **Recent meta-analysis of observational study** found no suggestion that vaginal estrogen impacts risk of breast cancer.

- **Endometrial safety – Cochrane Review 2009**
  In 6 – 24 months of vaginal oestrogen therapy, no endometrial hyperplasia, no progesterone supplement and therefore no endometrial surveillance required in asymptomatic, low risk women receiving estrogen in prescribed dose and duration of treatment.

Individual dose is 10 mcg/day and studies have found annual absorption of estradiol is only 1.14 mg. There are studies on long term risk of vaginal preparation use, but it is absolutely clear that absorption is negligible after atrophic changes are reversed.

Cancers and Local Vaginal Estrogen Therapy:

Local vaginal estrogen therapy is a cornerstone in managing Genitourinary Syndrome of Menopause (GSM), effectively alleviating symptoms such as vaginal dryness, irritation, and urinary discomfort. However, its use in individuals with a history of estrogen-dependent cancers, particularly breast cancer, necessitates careful consideration.

Limited data is available on the use of vaginal estrogen therapy in women with breast and endometrial cancer.

- Lifestyle modifications and nonhormonal treatment should be the first option.

- But in resistant or severe cases, vaginal estrogen may be used in lower doses after joint consultation with the oncologist.

- Counselling of women should be done before prescribing vaginal estrogen.

- Preferred therapy is low dose and low potency estrogen 'Estriol' where metabolic clearance is also rapid.

Systemic Hormone Therapy:

- **Systemic therapy is not indicated for GSM.**

- Urogenital symptoms associated with menopausal symptoms (especially severe vasomotor symptoms) is an indication for systemic hormone therapy to be combined with local vaginal therapy.

- Both systemic and local vaginal therapies can be given in combination where it is required and where there are no contraindications for systemic therapy as per the guidelines.

- It is estimated that approximately 25 % of women taking oral hormone therapy have persistent vaginal dryness and other urogenital symptoms. In such situations additional local estrogen therapy can be prescribed.

Tibolone:

- Systemic steroid having 2 estrogenic, 1 progestogenic and 1 androgenic metabolite.

- Used for prevention of vasomotor symptoms and bone loss. It has an additional advantage of improving **'libido and sexual desire'.**

- The clinical effects are due to the mild estrogenic action of delta-4-isomer, which reduces the SHBG level and increases the bioavailability of testosterone, estradiol and DHEA-S.

- Estrogenic effects on vagina decrease the vaginal dryness and decrease dyspareunia.

- The androgenic effect of tibolone helps to improve libido.

- The combined effects cause an overall improvement in mood, libido and sexual enjoyment thus improving quality of life.

- Dosage of tibolone is 2.5 mg orally/ day, even 1.25 mg / day has the same results.

Ospemifene:

- Ospemifene is the third generation SERM approved by FDA in 2013 in the treatment of moderate to severe dyspareunia due to vulvovaginal atrophy (VVA). Again, it is recently approved in 2019 for moderate to severe vaginal dryness as a symptom of VVA.

- Relative to other SERMs (e.g. Tamoxifen, Raloxifene, Bazedoxifene), Ospemifene has strong agonistic activity on vaginal tissues, antagonistic properties on breast tissue and weak partial and neutral activity on endometrial tissue.

- Ospemifene was initially developed for osteoporosis but has shown favourable oestrogenic effect on the vaginal epithelium with significant improvement in vaginal maturation index (VMI), vaginal ph and vaginal dryness.

- In a pilot study, ospemifene was shown to normalise vestibular innervation sensitivity, possibly through an anti-neuroinflammatory activity, which may explain its efficacy against symptoms of vaginal burning and introital dyspareunia.

- Although evidence is retrospective and patient numbers were small, treatment with ospemifene for 12 weeks for postmenopausal women with VVA and overactive bladder syndrome was associated with significant decrease in the number of voids, urgent micturition events.

- It is the only therapeutic option approved for the use in women with VVA with a history of breast cancer after all breast cancer treatment has been completed (Breast cancer survivors).

- Ospemifene is administered orally and therefore it avoids the inconveniences of administration of vaginal estrogen with some women.

- The typical dosing is 60 mg orally once daily. Half-life is 26 hrs. Mostly metabolised in liver, 75 % excreted in faeces, 7 % in urine as metabolites and minimal amount excreted unchanged in urine.

- Endometrial safety of adding progesterone to ospemifene therapy has not been evaluated clinically. Given all the available clinical data, ospemifene should be used as a single agent therapy without progesterone for the shortest possible period for approved indication with adequate clinical surveillance.

- The most frequently reported adverse effect is hot flashes. Other rare side effects include swelling or pain in legs, warm or red skin, dizziness, weakness. If such adverse effects develop, you first stop the treatment and visit your doctor for further advice.

Tissue Selective Estrogen Complexes (TSECs):

- These complexes are SERMs in combination with estrogen.

- Relieves hot flashes, treats VVA, prevents bone loss and has a protective effect on endometrium and breast.

- Bazedoxifene (BZA) paired with conjugated equine estrogen (CEE) is the first TSEC.

- BZA 20 mg / CEE 0.45 mg showed significant improvement in vaginal ph and VVA symptoms.

Dehydroepiandrosterone Acetate (DHEA) (Also known as Prasterone):

- Sex steroid precursor, shows good effect on sexual function.

- In 2016, FDA approved intravaginal Prasterone, a DHEA containing product for the treatment of dyspareunia secondary to moderate to severe vulvovaginal atrophy caused by oestrogen deficiency in menopause.

- The secretion of DHEA decreases with age, with an average 60 % decrease during menopause.

- A number of studies have shown that DHEA administered intravaginal over a 12 weeks period reduces vaginal pH, improves VMI with a better physical appearance of vagina.

- Recent data has shown the benefits of the local intravaginal action of DHEA on quality of life and all domains of sexual dysfunction, especially the most bothersome symptoms (dyspareunia and vaginal dryness) with an improvement of 41.3 % compared with placebo.

- Intravaginal DHEA acts on all three layers of vagina making it superior over intravaginal estrogen which acts mainly on the superficial epithelial layer.

- It induces mucification of the epithelium.

- Increases density of collagen fibres in the vaginal wall.

- Stimulates the muscle layer.

- Most common intravaginal dosage for DHEA is 6.5 mg daily for 12 weeks.

- Portman et.al. analysed the effects of DHEA on endometrium through biopsies at the end of 12 weeks of intravaginal therapy. The results showed atrophic or inactive endometrium, confirming its safety.

- Further studies are needed to support the use of intravaginal DHEA for postmenopausal women with vulvovaginal atrophy.

Phytoestrogens:

- Systemic phytoestrogens do not seem to have any effect on vaginal epithelium however local intravaginal phytoestrogen improves vaginal maturation index (VMI).

- In a study, 90 postmenopausal women were treated for 12 weeks with either isoflavone vaginal gel 4 % (1 gm /day), CEE cream (0.3 mg / day) or placebo gel. Women treated with isoflavone gel showed a similar improvement as in the estrogen group for vaginal dryness and dyspareunia. Both of which differed significantly from the placebo group. This study showed some promise.

- Many more such studies are necessary to make isoflavone vaginal gel as a viable option for women who have contraindications to vaginal oestrogen therapy.

- Isoflavone vaginal gel available in the market is Iseren gel.

Some of the preparations available in market for GSM:

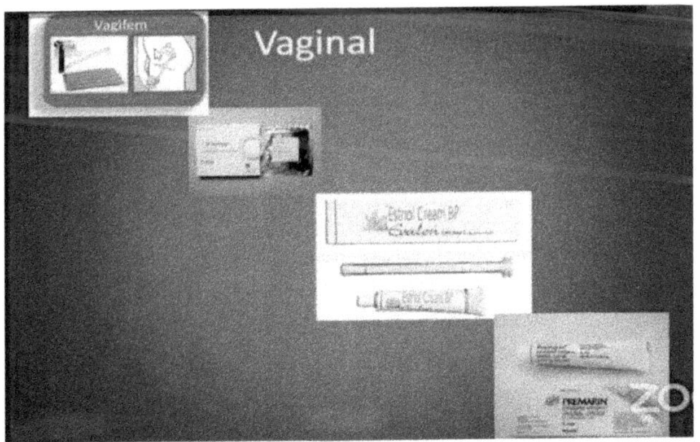

Phytoestrogens

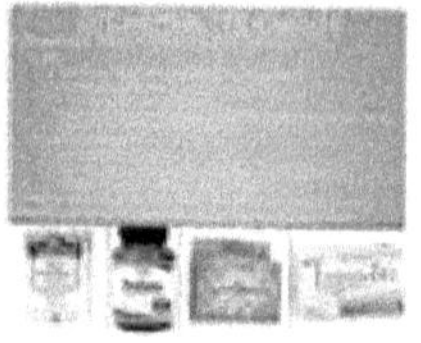

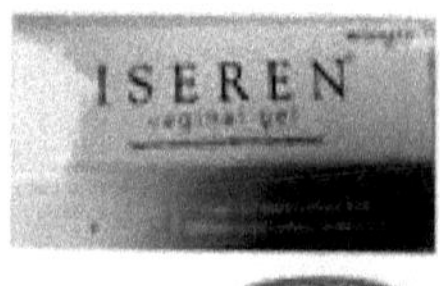

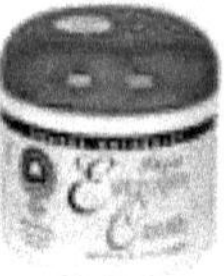

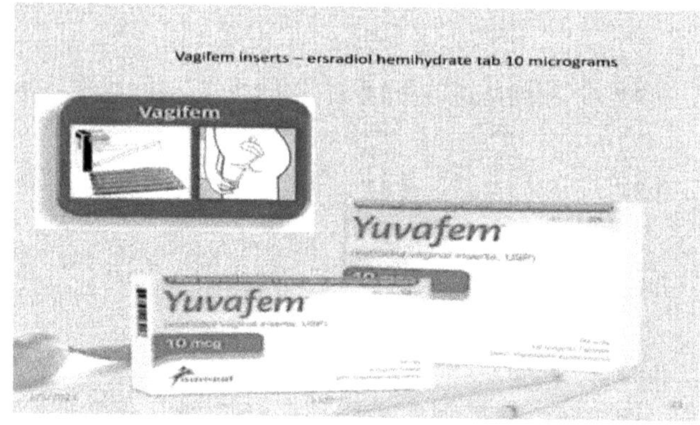

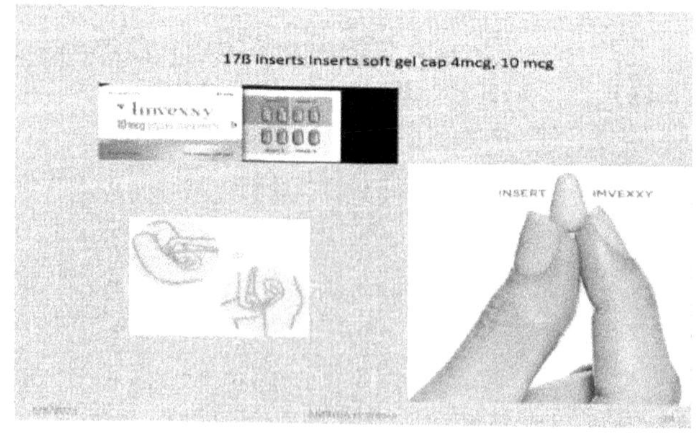

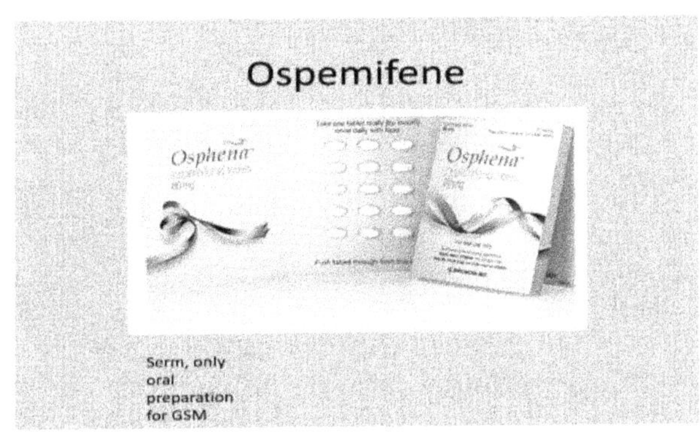
Ospemifene
Osphena
Osphena
Serm, only
oral
preparation
for GSM

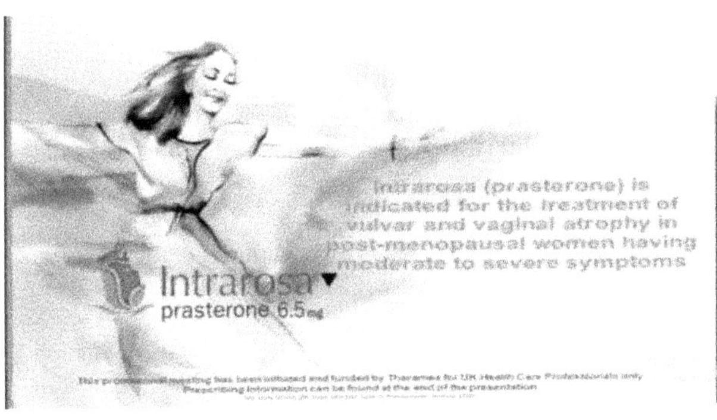
Intrarosa (prasterone) is
indicated for the treatment of
vulvar and vaginal atrophy in
post-menopausal women having
moderate to severe symptoms
Intrarosa▼
prasterone 6.5mg

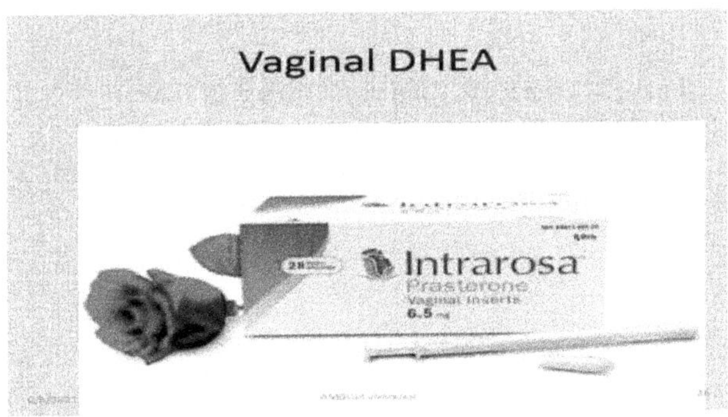
Vaginal DHEA
Intrarosa
Prasterone
Vaginal inserts
6.5 mg

Laser Therapy in Genitourinary Symptoms of Menopause (GSM)

Laser therapy has emerged as a promising non-hormonal treatment option for managing genitourinary symptoms of menopause (GSM). It provides relief by promoting collagen remodeling, restoring vaginal mucosa, and improving urogenital function. Long-term safety data is still evolving. Below are the main types of laser therapies and their usefulness:

Types of Laser Therapies:

- **Fractional CO_2 Laser (Carbon Dioxide Laser):**
  - **Mechanism:** Utilizes a controlled thermal effect to stimulate collagen production and enhance vaginal tissue elasticity.
  - **Usefulness:**
    - Improves vaginal dryness, atrophy, and elasticity.
    - Reduces dyspareunia (painful intercourse).
    - Relieves mild urinary symptoms like frequency and urgency.
    - Enhances vaginal mucosal integrity and hydration.
- **Er: YAG Laser (Erbium: Yttrium-Aluminum-Garnet):**
  - **Mechanism:** Delivers a non-ablative thermal effect to rejuvenate vaginal tissues with minimal downtime.
  - **Usefulness:**
    - Effective for treating vaginal dryness, irritation, and burning.
    - Improves symptoms of mild stress urinary incontinence.
    - Faster recovery compared to CO_2 laser.
    - Gentle on delicate vaginal tissues.

- **Nd: YAG Laser (Neodymium-Doped Yttrium-Aluminum-Garnet):**
  - **Mechanism:** Penetrates deeper layers of tissue to promote tissue remodeling and improve vascularity.
  - **Usefulness:**
    - Targets deeper layers of vaginal tissues for enhanced firmness.
    - Helps with stress urinary incontinence and pelvic laxity.
    - Less commonly used for GSM but beneficial in selected cases.

General Usefulness of Laser Therapy in GSM:

- **Non-Hormonal Option:**
  - Ideal for women contraindicated for hormonal treatments, such as those with a history of breast cancer or thromboembolism.
- **Minimally Invasive:**
  - Outpatient procedure with no need for anesthesia or significant downtime.
- **Improved Vaginal Health:**
  - Enhances epithelial thickness and lubrication.
  - Alleviates symptoms like dryness, itching, burning, and dyspareunia.
- **Pelvic Floor Support:**
  - Provides mild to moderate improvement in stress urinary incontinence and pelvic laxity.
- **Psychological and Quality of Life Improvement:**
  - Restores confidence and sexual satisfaction.
- **Durability of Results:**
  - Relief typically lasts 6–12 months, with maintenance sessions required.
- **Cautions and Limitations:**
  - **Not suitable** for severe prolapse or advanced urinary incontinence.
  - May require multiple sessions for optimal results and therefore the cost-effectiveness.

CHAPTER VII: MHT AND SPECIAL SITUATIONS

"Science is organized knowledge.

Wisdom is organized life."

– Immanuel Kant

(A) MHT And Breast Cancer Disease Risk

- Baseline risk of breast cancer for women around menopausal age varies from one woman to another depending on the underlying risk factors.

- MHT with estrogen and synthetic progesterone (Medroxyprogesterone Acetate MPA) which was used for women with intact uterus, was associated with a small increase in the risk of breast cancer.

- MHT with estrogen and progesterone (Micronized progesterone) definitely reduces the risk than MPA.

- MHT with estrogen alone which is used for hysterectomized women, is associated with little or no change in the baseline risk of breast cancer.

- Any risk associated with the baseline risk of breast cancer is related to the treatment duration and the type of progesterone. Large observational studies suggest that micronized progesterone and dydrogesterone may be associated with a lower risk of invasive breast cancer compared to synthetic progesterone including medroxyprogesterone acetate (MPA) if given for less than 5 years.

Key Studies on MHT Containing MPA and Breast Cancer Risk

- **Women's Health Initiative (WHI Study 1993-1998)**
  - **Study Design:** Large randomized controlled trial (RCT) involving over 16,000 postmenopausal women.

  - **Findings (2000):**
    - Use of **estrogen + MPA** was associated with a significant increase in breast cancer risk compared to placebo.
    - After 5.6 years of follow-up, the risk of invasive breast cancer was 24% higher in the combined MHT group.
    - Increased breast density observed, which may have implications for mammographic detection.
    - Risk persisted even after discontinuation of therapy, with a "lag effect" noted.

  - **Mechanisms:**
    - MPA appears to amplify estrogen's proliferative effects on breast tissue.
    - Induction of pro-inflammatory pathways and mitogenic signaling.

- **Million Women Study (MWS 2003)**
  - **Study Design:** Observational study involving over 1 million women in the UK.

  - **Findings:**
    - Combined MHT (estrogen + MPA) was linked to a significantly higher risk of breast cancer compared to estrogen-alone therapy.
    - Risk increased with longer duration of use:
    - Up to 2-fold increased risk with prolonged use (>5 years).
    - Risk diminished after discontinuation but remained elevated compared to non-users.

- **Nurses' Health Study (1980 to 1994)**
    - **Study Design:** Prospective cohort study using oral conjugated estrogens (CEE 0.625 mg/day) + MPA and following up to 2002.

    - **Findings:**
        - Long-term use (>10 years) of combined MHT with MPA was associated with a higher breast cancer incidence compared to short-term use (3 – 5 years).
        - Suggests a dose-response relationship between duration and risk.

- **E3N Cohort Study (France)**
    - **Study Design:** Observational study involving French women.

    - **Findings:**
        - MPA-containing MHT had a stronger association with breast cancer risk than regimens using micronized progesterone.
        - Suggests that the type of progestogen significantly impacts risk.

Evidence-Based Summary conclude that:

- There is robust evidence linking combined MHT with MPA to an increased risk of breast cancer.

- Risks are dose and duration-dependent and also the type of progesterone used in MHT, Micronized progesterone and Dydrogesterone showing a potentially safer profile.

- Further research is needed to explore safer hormonal options and redefine guidelines for personalized therapy.

The increased risk due to MHT is similar or lower than those associated with lifestyle factors such as:

- Sedentary lifestyle
- Obesity
- Excessive alcohol consumption
- Cigarette smoking

Based on the UK data, things are very clear in the table below:

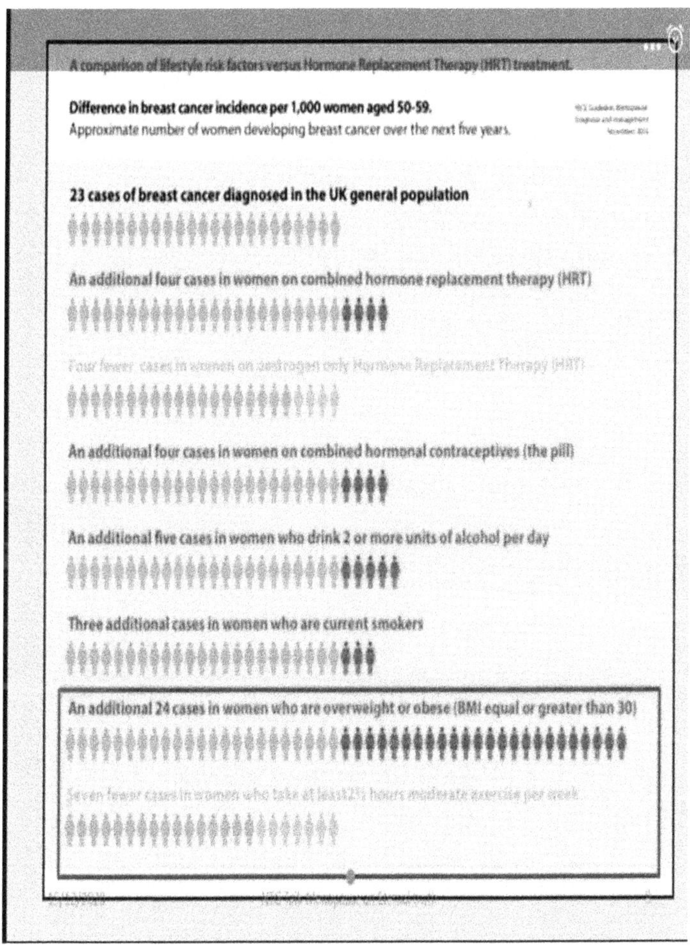

(B) MHT And Cardiovascular Disease Risk

Introduction

- **Cardiovascular Disease (CVD)**: A leading cause of morbidity and mortality among postmenopausal women.

- **Role of MHT**: Initially thought to protect against CVD due to estrogen's favorable effects on lipids and vasodilation. However, early studies challenged this assumption, showing varied effects depending on age, timing of initiation, and type of MHT.

Key Initial Studies on MHT and CVD Risk

- **Women's Health Initiative (WHI) Study (1990s)**
    - **Study Design**:
        - Randomized Controlled Trial (RCT) examining MHT in postmenopausal women aged 50–79 years.
    - **Findings**:
        - **Combined MHT (Estrogen + Progestogen)**:
            - ✓ Increased risk of coronary heart disease (CHD) within the first year of use.
            - ✓ Increased risk of stroke and venous thromboembolism (VTE).
        - **Estrogen-only MHT** (in women without a uterus):
            - ✓ No significant increase in CHD risk.
            - ✓ Increased risk of stroke.
            - ✓ Protective effects were not observed in older women (mean age: 63 years).
        - **Implication**: MHT was initially contraindicated for CVD prevention.

- **Heart and Estrogen/Progestin Replacement Study (HERS)**
    - **Study Design**:
        - RCT in women with existing coronary artery disease (secondary prevention).
    - **Findings**:
        - No reduction in recurrent CVD events with MHT.
        - Early increase in thrombotic events and no overall benefit.
    - **Evolution of Understanding: The "Timing Hypothesis"**
        - Subsequent analyses proposed that the **timing of MHT initiation** is critical:
        - **Younger Postmenopausal Women (Age <60, Within 10 Years of Menopause):**
        - Possible cardioprotective effects due to estrogen's ability to maintain endothelial function, improve lipid profile, and reduce vascular inflammation.
        - **Older Women or Late Initiation (Age >60, >10 Years After Menopause):**
        - Adverse effects likely due to existing atherosclerotic plaques and prothrombotic tendencies.
- **Current Recommendations Based on Updated Evidence Risk Stratification**
    - **Assess Baseline CVD Risk:**
        - History of coronary artery disease, stroke, or thromboembolism.
        - Presence of risk factors: hypertension, diabetes, dyslipidemia, smoking, obesity.
        - Use risk calculators like ASCVD risk score.
    - **Individualized Decision-Making:**
        - Weigh benefits of MHT for menopausal symptoms against CVD risks.

- MHT is not recommended for primary or secondary prevention of CVD.

- **Choice of MHT**
  Estrogen-Only MHT:
  - Safer for CVD risk in women without a uterus.
  - Transdermal estrogen may lower VTE risk compared to oral formulations.

- **Combined MHT (Estrogen + Progestogen)**:
  - Use micronized progesterone or dydrogesterone, which have a lower risk profile compared to synthetic progestins like medroxyprogesterone acetate (MPA).

- **Route of Administration**:
  - **Transdermal MHT**: Avoids first-pass metabolism, reducing risks of VTE, stroke, and hypertriglyceridemia.
  - **Oral MHT**: Higher risks of thrombotic events and hepatic effects.

- **Timing and Duration**
  - Start MHT **within 10 years of menopause onset** or before age 60, if indicated.
  - Use the **lowest effective dose** for the **shortest duration** needed to manage symptoms.
  - Reassess annually to evaluate the need for continued therapy.

- **Monitoring and Follow-Up**
  - Regular monitoring of blood pressure, lipids, and glucose.
  - Encourage a heart-healthy lifestyle.

- **In Summary:**
  - Initial studies like WHI and HERS highlighted the potential cardiovascular risks of MHT, leading to significant changes in clinical guidelines.

    - The "timing hypothesis" has refined the understanding of when and how to use MHT safely.
    - MHT should not be used for CVD prevention, but careful patient selection and individualized treatment can minimize risks and provide symptom relief.

Menopause Hormone Therapy (MHT) cannot be used for the primary or secondary prevention of cardiovascular disease (CVD) is supported by evidence from major studies.

- **Women's Health Initiative (WHI) Study**:
  - **Combined MHT (Estrogen + Progestogen):**
    - Increased risk of coronary heart disease (CHD) in older women (>10 years postmenopause).
    - Increased risk of stroke and venous thromboembolism (VTE).

  - **Estrogen-Only Therapy** (in women without a uterus):
    - Neutral effect on CHD risk, but an increased risk of stroke.
    - Conclusion: MHT does not reduce the risk of CVD in postmenopausal women and may increase risks when initiated late.

  - **Pathophysiological Considerations**
    - While estrogen improves endothelial function and lipid profiles in younger women, its effects on existing atherosclerotic plaques in older women can destabilize plaques, leading to thrombotic events.

- **HERS Trial**:
  - Showed no reduction in recurrent CHD events in women with established coronary artery disease.

  - Increased risk of CHD events in the first year of MHT use.

- **Meta-Analyses**:
  Consistently demonstrate that MHT does not reduce CVD risk in women with pre-existing conditions and may exacerbate risks in some cases.

- **Mechanistic Explanation**
  MHT, particularly oral formulations, increases the risk of:
  - Thromboembolic events due to enhanced clotting factor production.
  - Stroke due to pro-inflammatory and pro-thrombotic effects on vulnerable plaques.
  - In women with established CVD, these mechanisms counteract the potential vasodilatory and anti-inflammatory benefits of estrogen.

In Summary:

- **Primary Prevention**: MHT does not reduce the risk of developing CVD and may increase risks when initiated late in menopause. Non-hormonal interventions should be prioritized for CVD prevention.

- **Secondary Prevention**: MHT is contraindicated for women with established CVD, as evidence shows no benefit and potential harm.

- **MHT should not be used for cardiovascular disease prevention—neither primary nor secondary.** Its role should be confined to alleviating menopausal symptoms such as severe vasomotor symptoms, with a careful, individualized approach that considers timing, formulation, and overall risk profile. MHT may be cardio protective, if started in perimenopause or early postmenopause for VMS in healthy women. It reduces the risk of type II diabetes and has positive effect on the lipid profile and metabolic syndrome.

(C) MHT In Managing Vasomotor Symptoms in Women with Type II Diabetes

Diabetes is a common comorbidity in postmenopausal women, and the hormonal changes of menopause can exacerbate insulin resistance and cardiovascular risks. Menopause Hormone Therapy (MHT) offers relief for menopausal symptoms and potential metabolic benefits. However, its use in women with diabetes requires careful evaluation and a personalized approach.

- **Benefits of MHT in Diabetes:**
  - **Improved Glycemic Control:**
    Estrogen enhances insulin sensitivity by improving hepatic and peripheral glucose metabolism.

  - **Reduction in Visceral Adiposity:**
    MHT helps decrease central obesity, reducing the risk of metabolic syndrome.

  - **Cardioprotective Effects:**
    MHT improves lipid profiles (e.g., raising HDL, reducing LDL), mitigating cardiovascular risks associated with diabetes.

- **Risks Associated with MHT in Diabetes:**
  - **Thromboembolic Events:**
    Women with diabetes are at a higher baseline risk for thromboembolism, which may be further increased by certain MHT formulations.

  - **Progestogen-Related Effects:**
    Some progestogens may worsen insulin resistance, necessitating careful selection of the type and dose.

- **Weight and Hyperglycemia:**
  Monitoring is essential, as some women may experience weight gain or altered glycemic control.

- **Preferred Treatment Strategies:**
  - **Formulation Choice:**
    - **Transdermal Estrogen:** A safer option as it avoids first-pass hepatic metabolism, minimizing impacts on glucose metabolism and coagulation pathways.
    - **Micronized Progesterone/Dydrogesterone:** These options are metabolically neutral compared to synthetic progestogens.

  - **Early Initiation:**
    - Starting MHT within 10 years of menopause or before the age of 60 enhances benefits and minimizes risks.

  - **Monitoring and Duration:**
    - Regular follow-ups to assess glucose levels, lipid profiles, and cardiovascular health are critical.
    - Use the lowest effective dose for the shortest necessary duration.

- **Clinical Guidelines for MHT in Diabetes:**
  - **Assessment:** Comprehensive evaluation of cardiovascular, thromboembolic, and metabolic risks before initiation.

  - **Lifestyle Integration:** Encourage dietary adjustments, physical activity, and weight management alongside MHT.

In Summary:

- **Avoid MHT in Women with:**
  - Poorly controlled diabetes
  - Active cardiovascular disease,
  - History of thromboembolism or breast cancer.

- **MHT can be prescribed for symptomatic relief:**
  - Perimenopausal
  - Recently postmenopausal
  - Low risk CVD

(D) MHT For Managing Vasomotor Symptoms in Women with Hypertension

Hypertension is prevalent in postmenopausal women, and the hormonal changes during menopause may exacerbate vascular dysfunction and elevate blood pressure. While MHT offers symptom relief and potential cardiovascular benefits, its use in hypertensive women must be tailored to minimize risks and maximize therapeutic outcomes.

Effects of MHT on Blood Pressure

- **Estrogen's Role:**
  - **Favorable Effects:** Estrogen improves endothelial function, promotes vasodilation by increasing nitric oxide availability, and reduces arterial stiffness.

  - **Potential Concerns:** Oral estrogens may increase renin substrate levels, leading to slight elevations in blood pressure in some women.

- **Progestogens:**
  - Certain synthetic progestogens may negate the vasodilatory effects of estrogen or worsen blood pressure. Micronized progesterone is preferable for its neutral vascular effects.

Preferred Approach to MHT in Hypertensive Women

- **Formulation Selection:**
  - **Transdermal Estrogen:** This is the recommended route for hypertensive women. It bypasses the liver, avoiding first-pass metabolism, and has minimal impact on blood pressure.

  - Transdermal estrogen has been shown to have a **neutral or even lowering effect on blood pressure** in postmenopausal women. (**Reference:** Scuteri et al., *Hypertension*, 2012)

  - **Micronized Progesterone or Dydrogesterone:** These are preferred over synthetic progestins for their safer cardiovascular profiles. (**Reference:** Canonico et al., *European Heart Journal*, 2014).

- **Dose and Timing:**
  - Use the lowest effective dose to alleviate symptoms.

  - **Study:** The **Early vs. Late Intervention Trial with Estradiol (ELITE)** explored the timing of MHT initiation. (**Reference:** Hodis et al., *New England Journal of Medicine*, 2016).

  - **Findings:**
    - MHT initiated within 6 years of menopause reduced carotid intima-media thickness progression, suggesting vascular benefits.
    - Women with controlled hypertension benefited from the cardiovascular protective effects of MHT.

- **Clinical Monitoring:**
  - **Baseline Assessment:**
    Conduct a thorough evaluation of blood pressure, lipid profile, and overall cardiovascular risk.

- **Follow-Up:**
  - Monitor blood pressure at regular intervals after initiating MHT.
  - Adjust therapy if significant blood pressure elevations occur.
- **Contraindications:**
  - **Avoid MHT in women with:**
    - Untreated / Uncontrolled hypertension.
    - Hypertensive heart disease or advanced cardiovascular complications.
    - A history of stroke or thromboembolic events.

(E) MHT And VTE

- The risk of VTE increases with age especially after 45 years of age.
- The risk of VTE is increased by smoking, increasing age, obesity and oral MHT.
- VTE risk is as high as 29/10000 women-years during pregnancy and 300-400/10000 women-years in postpartum period.
- WHI observational study revealed a lower risk in those not exposed to MHT (1.6/1000 women-years) while it showed a higher rate (2.4/1000 women-years) in those exposed to MHT.
- Oral MHT preparations increase risk by 2-4-fold. Risk is highest in the first year of use. Transdermal preparations are associated with lower risk.

- Evidence from observational studies suggest that micronized progesterone and dydrogesterone may be associated with a lower risk of VTE compared to synthetic progesterone like DMA.

- MHT is contraindicated in women with history of VTE.

(F) MHT Use in Women with POI (Premature Ovarian Insufficiency)

Premature Ovarian Insufficiency (POI), characterized by the loss of ovarian function before the age of 40, presents unique challenges in women's health. It is distinct from natural menopause due to the younger age of onset and the significant long-term impact on physical and emotional well-being. Menopause Hormone Therapy (MHT) is considered a cornerstone in the management of POI to mitigate these effects. Below are key aspects to consider:

Importance of MHT in POI:

- **Physiological Hormone Replacement**: MHT restores hormone levels closer to physiological levels, helping to mimic natural ovarian function.

- **Prevention of Long-Term Health Risks**:
  - **Bone Health**: Reduced estrogen in POI accelerates bone loss, increasing the risk of osteoporosis and fractures. MHT helps maintain bone mineral density (BMD).

  - **Cardiovascular Protection**: Estrogen deficiency is linked to an increased risk of cardiovascular diseases. Early MHT initiation reduces this risk.

- **Neuroprotection**: MHT may offer protection against cognitive decline and neurodegenerative diseases such as Alzheimer's.

- **Quality of Life**: Improves symptoms like hot flashes, mood swings, sexual dysfunction, and sleep disturbances.

Selection of Therapy:

- **Hormonal Components**:
  - **Estrogen**: Estradiol is preferred for systemic benefits, administered transdermal or orally.

  - **Progesterone**: Added to protect the endometrium in women with an intact uterus. Micronized progesterone is often favored for its minimal side effects.

- **Mode of Delivery**:
  - **Transdermal Estrogen**: Reduces risks associated with oral estrogen, such as venous thromboembolism (VTE) and liver metabolism.

  - **Combined Oral Contraceptives (COCs)**: Sometimes used in younger women for cycle regulation and contraceptive benefits, though they may not fully address long-term health risks.

Duration and Monitoring:

- **Duration**: MHT in women with POI is recommended until the average age of natural menopause (around 50 years), after which risks and benefits of continued therapy should be reassessed.

Monitoring:

- Regular assessment of BMD via DEXA scans.

- Cardiovascular health monitoring (lipid profile, blood pressure).
- Symptom evaluation and therapy adjustment.

Contraindications and Precautions:

- **Absolute Contraindications**: Active or history of hormone-sensitive cancers, unexplained vaginal bleeding, thromboembolic disorders.
- **Relative Contraindications**: Requires individual assessment, including conditions like uncontrolled hypertension or liver disease.

Psychosocial Aspects:

- Women with POI may experience psychological distress, infertility concerns, and altered body image. MHT can contribute to psychological well-being by alleviating symptoms and restoring a sense of normalcy.

Research and Advances:

- Emerging therapies, including selective estrogen receptor modulators (SERMs) and tissue-selective estrogen complexes, may offer future options for POI management.
- Focus on personalized medicine ensures therapy is tailored based on genetic, metabolic, and symptomatic profiles.

In summary, MHT plays a critical role in the management of POI by addressing both short- and long-term health consequences of estrogen deficiency. A tailored approach, considering the individual patient's symptoms, risk factors, and preferences, is essential for optimal outcomes. Early initiation and appropriate monitoring ensure benefits of MHT.

(G) MHT And Early Onset Menopause

Menopause Hormone Therapy (MHT) plays a critical role in managing symptoms and health risks associated with **early-onset menopause** (menopause occurring between the age of 40 and the natural age of menopause, typically around 50–52 years). Here are key aspects to consider:

Challenges of Early-Onset Menopause:

- Early-onset menopause may result from **natural causes**, **surgical removal of ovaries**, **chemotherapy/radiation**, or **genetic factors**. Women experiencing early menopause are at an increased risk of:
    - **Vasomotor symptoms** (hot flashes, night sweats).
    - **Urogenital atrophy** (vaginal dryness, painful intercourse).
    - **Osteoporosis** (due to decreased bone density from estrogen deficiency).
    - **Cardiovascular risks** (due to altered lipid profiles and vascular health).
    - **Cognitive decline** and mood disorders, including depression.

Benefits of MHT for Early-Onset Menopause:

MHT is the cornerstone of treatment for women with early menopause, especially those under the age of 45, as it helps prevent long-term complications associated with estrogen deficiency:

Relief of Symptoms:

- Effectively manages vasomotor symptoms.
- Improves sleep quality and overall quality of life.

- **Bone Health:**
  Reduces the risk of osteoporosis and fractures by maintaining bone density.

- **Cardiovascular Health:**
  Offers protective effects on lipid profiles, vascular function, and heart health.

- **Cognitive Benefits:**
  Helps in maintaining cognitive function and reducing risks of Alzheimer's disease in some cases.

- **Psychological Well-being:**
  Reduces anxiety, depression, and mood swings linked to hormonal changes.

MHT Regimens for Early-Onset Menopause:

- **Estrogen Therapy:**
  Recommended for women without a uterus (e.g., after hysterectomy).

- **Estrogen-Progestogen Therapy (EPT):**
  Used for women with an intact uterus to prevent endometrial hyperplasia and cancer.

- **Transdermal MHT:**
  Preferred in women with cardiovascular risk factors or liver dysfunction, as it bypasses hepatic metabolism.

Duration and Timing of MHT

- For women with early-onset menopause, MHT is typically continued **until the average age of natural menopause** (around 50–52 years).

- Long-term use beyond this age should be evaluated based on **individual risks** and **benefits**.

Special Considerations:

- **Contraindications:** Women with a history of breast cancer, thromboembolic events, or active liver disease should be carefully assessed.
- **Individualization:** Therapy should be tailored based on the woman's symptoms, risks, and preferences.
- **Non-Hormonal Options:** For women unable to take MHT, alternative therapies (e.g., SSRIs, SNRIs, or bone-specific medications) may be considered.

Monitoring and Follow-Up:

- Regular follow-up is essential to monitor symptoms, adjust dosages, and assess risks.
- Focus on bone density testing, cardiovascular health, and cancer screenings.

In summary, MHT provides significant health benefits for women experiencing early-onset menopause. Its role extends beyond symptom management to preventing long-term complications like osteoporosis, cardiovascular disease, and cognitive decline. Careful assessment and individualized treatment plans ensure that the therapy is both safe and effective.

(H) MHT And Medically Induced Menopause

Medically induced menopause occurs when ovarian function is lost due to **medical interventions** such as chronic treatments with corticosteroids, chemotherapy, radiation therapy, or surgical removal of ovaries. The abrupt decline in estrogen levels can lead to severe symptoms and long-term health risks, making **Menopause Hormone Therapy (MHT)** a crucial component of management.

Causes of Medically Induced Menopause:

- **Chronic Corticosteroid Use:**
    - Long-term corticosteroid therapy can suppress hypothalamic-pituitary-ovarian (HPO) axis function, leading to ovarian insufficiency and eventual menopause.
    - Conditions requiring high-dose corticosteroids, such as systemic lupus erythematosus (SLE), rheumatoid arthritis, or inflammatory bowel disease (IBD), often predispose patients to earlier ovarian dysfunction.
    - Coexisting conditions such as diabetes, thyroid disorders, or previous ovarian damage (e.g., chemotherapy or pelvic radiation) increase risk.
    - **High-dose corticosteroids** (e.g., prednisone ≥7.5–10 mg/day or equivalent) taken chronically have the greatest impact on ovarian function.
    - Even **moderate doses** (5–7.5 mg/day) over an extended period can lead to HPO axis suppression.
    - Long-term use (≥6 months) of corticosteroids increases the likelihood of ovarian suppression.

    - Short-term use or intermittent corticosteroid therapy is less likely to cause menopause.

    - **Cumulative Effect:**
      The total cumulative dose is critical. For example, a **prednisone-equivalent dose >5 grams over a lifetime** has been associated with ovarian dysfunction.

    - Long-acting corticosteroids (e.g., dexamethasone) may have a more pronounced effect than shorter-acting options.

- **Chemotherapy and Radiation:**
  Cytotoxic agents and radiation can damage ovarian follicles, leading to premature ovarian failure.

- **Surgical Oophorectomy:**
  The surgical removal of ovaries immediately induces menopause.

- **Other Medications:**
  GnRH agonists/antagonists used in endometriosis or cancer treatment may induce menopause temporarily or permanently.

Symptoms and Risks:

Medically induced menopause often causes **more severe and abrupt symptoms** than natural menopause due to the sudden drop in estrogen levels:

- **Acute Symptoms:**
    - Intense vasomotor symptoms (hot flashes, night sweats).

    - Severe urogenital atrophy (vaginal dryness, painful intercourse, urinary symptoms).

- Psychological effects (depression, anxiety, mood swings).

- **Long-Term Risks:**
  - Osteoporosis and fractures.
  - Cardiovascular diseases (due to unfavorable lipid profiles and vascular changes).
  - Cognitive decline and neurodegenerative risks.
  - Increased risk of metabolic syndrome.

- **Role of MHT in Medically Induced Menopause:** MHT is the primary treatment for managing symptoms and reducing long-term health risks in women with medically induced menopause.
  - **Benefits of MHT**
    - **Symptom Relief:** Effectively reduces vasomotor symptoms and improves quality of life.
    - **Bone Health:** Prevents rapid bone loss and reduces the risk of fractures.
    - **Cardiovascular Protection:** Maintains vascular health and lipid profiles, lowering cardiovascular risks.
    - **Urogenital Benefits:** Restores vaginal health and alleviates urinary symptoms.
    - **Mood and Cognitive Support:** Improves mood, reduces depression, and may help preserve cognitive function.
  - **Types of MHT:**
    - **Estrogen-Only Therapy (ET):** Recommended for women who have undergone hysterectomy.

- **Estrogen-Progestogen Therapy (EPT):** Used for women with an intact uterus to prevent endometrial hyperplasia.
- **Transdermal MHT:** Preferred in women at risk for thromboembolism or with liver dysfunction.

- **Timing and Duration of MHT**
  - **Early Initiation:** Starting MHT soon after medically induced menopause provides maximum benefits, particularly for cardiovascular and bone health.
  - **Duration:** Therapy is generally recommended until the average age of natural menopause (50–52 years). Continuation beyond this age should be individualized based on risks and benefits.

- **Special Considerations**
  - **Individualized Approach:** Therapy should be tailored based on the cause of menopause, age, symptoms, and risk factors.

- **Non-Hormonal Alternatives:**
  - Women with contraindications to MHT (e.g., breast cancer, thromboembolic disorders) may benefit from SSRIs, SNRIs, gabapentin, or clonidine for symptom relief.
  - Bisphosphonates or selective estrogen receptor modulators (SERMs) can be used for bone health.

- **Monitoring:** Regular follow-ups are essential to adjust therapy, monitor bone density, and assess cardiovascular and metabolic health.

In summary, medically induced menopause requires an integrated approach to manage symptoms and prevent long-term complications. MHT provides significant benefits, especially when initiated early.

(I) MHT Use in Women with Migraine with or without Aura

The use of Menopause Hormone Therapy (MHT) in women with migraines, particularly in those with aura, requires a nuanced approach due to the potential risks and benefits. Migraine, being hormonally influenced in many women, can be exacerbated or alleviated by hormone therapy depending on the type, formulation, and method of administration.

Migraine Types and Hormonal Influence:

- **Migraine Without Aura**: Generally considered safer for MHT. Symptoms may improve or remain stable during therapy.
- **Migraine With Aura**: Involves a higher baseline risk for ischemic stroke. Estrogen therapy, particularly oral formulations, may exacerbate this risk, necessitating careful consideration.

Key Considerations for MHT in Migraine:

- **Safety First**: In women with migraines, especially those with aura, the choice of therapy should focus on minimizing the risk of stroke and cardiovascular events.
- **Migraine Symptoms**: MHT may have variable effects on migraines:
    - **Improvement**: Stabilizing estrogen levels through therapy can reduce the frequency and severity of migraines in some women.

- **Exacerbation**: Fluctuating hormone levels or high doses of estrogen may worsen symptoms.

Recommendations for MHT in Women with Migraine:

- **Preferred MHT Formulation**:
  - **Transdermal Estrogen**: Low-dose transdermal estrogen (patch, gel, or spray) is recommended as it avoids first-pass metabolism and minimizes thromboembolic risk, which is critical in migraine with aura.
  - **Micronized Progesterone**: In women with an intact uterus, micronized progesterone is preferred due to its safer profile for migraines.

Avoid High-Dose Estrogen:

- High-dose oral estrogen increases stroke risk and can trigger migraines.
- Fluctuating hormone levels in oral therapy may exacerbate migraines.

Combination Therapy:

- In women requiring progesterone, avoid synthetic progestins as they may aggravate migraine symptoms; micronized progesterone is better tolerated.

Migraine With Aura and Stroke Risk:

- **Increased Baseline Risk**: Migraine with aura is an independent risk factor for ischemic stroke, further amplified by oral estrogen therapy.

- **Non-Oral Routes**: Transdermal estrogen has not been shown to significantly increase stroke risk and is preferred.

- **Lifestyle and Risk Management**: Women with migraine with aura should also optimize other stroke risk factors (e.g., avoid smoking, control hypertension, maintain a healthy weight).

Monitoring and Follow-Up:

- **Migraine Tracking**: Patients should maintain a headache diary to monitor the frequency and severity of migraines after initiating MHT.

- **Individualized Dosing**: Start with the lowest effective dose of estrogen and adjust based on symptom relief and migraine response.

- **Cardiovascular Monitoring**: Regular assessment of cardiovascular health is essential, especially in those with aura.

Alternatives to Estrogen Therapy:

For women with migraines where MHT is contraindicated or not well-tolerated:

- **Non-Hormonal Options**:
  - SSRIs or SNRIs for mood and vasomotor symptoms.
  - Gabapentin or clonidine for hot flashes.

- **Lifestyle Modifications**:
  - Regular sleep, hydration, and avoidance of known migraine triggers.
  - Magnesium and riboflavin supplementation may benefit some patients.

Special Scenarios:

- **Perimenopause**: Hormonal fluctuations in this phase may worsen migraines; continuous transdermal therapy can help stabilize hormone levels.

- **Postmenopause**: The decision to continue MHT should weigh the long-term benefits against stroke and cardiovascular risks, particularly in migraine with aura.

In Summary, in women with migraines, especially those with aura, MHT requires a cautious and individualized approach. Low-dose transdermal estrogen is the preferred option to stabilize hormone levels while minimizing vascular risks. Close monitoring and collaboration with a neurologist are crucial to safely managing symptoms and improving quality of life.

(J) MHT Use in Women with Breast Cancer Survivor

Menopause Hormone Therapy (MHT) in breast cancer survivors is a highly nuanced topic due to concerns about the potential for cancer recurrence. Estrogen and progesterone, which form the basis of MHT, may promote the growth of hormone-sensitive breast cancers. Consequently, MHT is generally avoided in this population unless there are exceptional circumstances. Below are critical considerations and recommendations for managing menopausal symptoms in breast cancer survivors:

General Considerations

- **Safety Concerns**: MHT, particularly systemic estrogen and progestogens, is typically contraindicated in breast cancer survivors, especially for hormone receptor-positive cancers.

- **Symptom Burden**: Many breast cancer survivors experience severe vasomotor symptoms (hot flashes, night sweats) and genitourinary syndrome of menopause (vaginal dryness, dyspareunia) that significantly impact quality of life.

- **Individualized Approach**: Therapy decisions should balance symptom management with the risk of recurrence, considering patient preferences and cancer characteristics.

Non-Hormonal Management of Menopausal Symptoms:

- **Vasomotor Symptoms**:
  - **First-Line Options**:
    - **Selective Serotonin Reuptake Inhibitors (SSRIs)** and **Selective Norepinephrine Reuptake Inhibitors (SNRIs)**: Examples include venlafaxine, paroxetine, or escitalopram.
    - **Gabapentin**: Effective for hot flashes, particularly at night.
    - **Clonidine**: May help reduce vasomotor symptoms but is less effective than SSRIs or SNRIs.

  - **Lifestyle Modifications**:
    - Regular physical activity.
    - Avoidance of known triggers (e.g., caffeine, alcohol, spicy foods).
    - Relaxation techniques like yoga, meditation, and paced breathing.

  - **Genitourinary Symptoms**:
    - **Non-Hormonal Vaginal Moisturizers and Lubricants**: For vaginal dryness and dyspareunia.
    - **Low-Dose Vaginal Estrogen**: Considered cautiously in some cases of severe symptoms if systemic absorption is minimal and oncologists are involved in decision-making.
    - **DHEA Vaginal Inserts (Prasterone)**: May improve local symptoms without significant systemic effects.

MHT Considerations in Exceptional Cases:

- **When MHT May Be Considered**:
    - Severe, refractory menopausal symptoms unresponsive to non-hormonal treatments.
    - Informed consent after thorough discussion of potential risks.

- **Preferred MHT Approach**:
    - Use of **ultra-low-dose transdermal estrogen** combined with local vaginal estrogen if necessary.
    - Avoid synthetic progestogens; micronized progesterone is a safer alternative if needed.

- **Collaboration with Oncologists**:
    - A multidisciplinary approach is crucial.
    - Treatment should be carefully documented and involve shared decision-making with the patient.

- **Risk Factors for Breast Cancer Recurrence:**
    - Before initiating MHT, evaluate:
        - **Cancer Type**: Hormone receptor-positive cancers pose higher risks.
        - **Recurrence Risk**: Consider tumor grade, nodal involvement, and response to initial treatment.
        - **Other Factors**: Age, time since cancer diagnosis, and co-existing comorbidities.

- **Emerging Therapies and Alternatives:**
    - **Tissue-Selective Estrogen Complexes (TSECs)**: Under investigation; potential to provide benefits without increasing breast tissue stimulation.
    - **Lifestyle and Complementary Therapies**: Weight loss, dietary changes, acupuncture, and cognitive behavioral therapy (CBT) may alleviate symptoms.
    - **Psychological and Emotional Support** Breast cancer survivors often face heightened anxiety about recurrence. Counseling and support groups can

play an important role in managing emotional and psychological challenges associated with menopause.

In summary, MHT is generally avoided in breast cancer survivors due to the potential risk of recurrence, particularly in hormone receptor-positive cases. Non-hormonal therapies and lifestyle modifications should be the first-line approach for managing menopausal symptoms. In exceptional cases, MHT may be cautiously considered with informed consent and close collaboration between the patient, oncologist, and gynecologist. A patient-centered, multidisciplinary approach is essential to ensure the best outcomes for symptom relief and cancer survivorship.

(K) MHT Use in Women with Fibroid Uterus

The use of Menopause Hormone Therapy (MHT) in women with uterine fibroids requires careful consideration of the potential effects of estrogen and progesterone on fibroid growth and related symptoms. While fibroids are non-cancerous growths that typically shrink after menopause due to declining estrogen levels, the introduction of exogenous hormones through MHT can influence their behavior.

Key Considerations:

- **Fibroid Growth**: Estrogen is a growth-promoting factor for fibroids, and MHT may stimulate their growth or prevent their postmenopausal regression.

- **Symptom Recurrence**: MHT may exacerbate symptoms such as abnormal uterine bleeding, pelvic pain, or pressure if fibroids increase in size.

- **Balance of Benefits and Risks**: The decision to use MHT depends on the severity of menopausal symptoms, the size and location of the fibroids, and the presence of symptoms related to the fibroids.

Recommendations for MHT in Women with Fibroids:

- **Preferred MHT Formulations**:
  Transdermal Estrogen:
  - Use the lowest effective dose to minimize systemic estrogen effects.
  - Transdermal formulations bypass first-pass metabolism, reducing the potential stimulation of fibroid growth.

- **Micronized Progesterone**:
  - For women with an intact uterus, micronized progesterone is preferred as it has a more favorable safety and tolerability profile compared to synthetic progestins.

- **Levonorgestrel-Releasing Intrauterine System (LNG-IUS)**:
  - Provides localized progestogenic effect, protects the endometrium, and may help control abnormal uterine bleeding associated with fibroids.

- **Avoidance of High-Dose Estrogen**:
  - High-dose systemic estrogen may significantly increase fibroid size or bleeding.

Monitoring and Adjustments:

- **Baseline Assessment**:
  - Perform a pelvic ultrasound to evaluate fibroid size, location, and symptoms before initiating MHT.

  - Rule out malignancy or other structural abnormalities that may mimic fibroids.

- **Regular Follow-Up**:
  - Monitor fibroid size and uterine bleeding during therapy.

  - Adjust MHT dose or discontinue therapy if significant fibroid-related symptoms develop.

- **Symptom Management**:
  - If fibroid-related symptoms recur, consider additional treatments such as:
    - Non-hormonal therapies for menopausal symptoms.
    - GnRH agonists or antagonists to reduce fibroid size temporarily.

Alternatives to Systemic MHT:

- For women with symptomatic fibroids or those at higher risk of fibroid growth:
  - **Non-Hormonal Therapies**:
    SSRIs/SNRIs, gabapentin, or clonidine for vasomotor symptoms.

  - **Lifestyle Modifications**:
    Regular exercise, a healthy diet, and weight management.

  - **Surgical Options**:
    If fibroids are causing significant symptoms, surgical options such as myomectomy, hysteroscopic resection, or even hysterectomy may be considered before initiating MHT.

Fibroids and Postmenopausal Bleeding:

- MHT users with a history of fibroids are at increased risk of postmenopausal bleeding, which warrants immediate evaluation to exclude endometrial hyperplasia or malignancy.

- If persistent bleeding occurs, consider discontinuing MHT or modifying the regimen.

Benefits vs. Risks of MHT in Fibroid Uterus:

- **Benefits**:
  - Relief from vasomotor symptoms, genitourinary syndrome of menopause, and improved quality of life.
  - Potential protection against osteoporosis and cardiovascular disease.
- **Risks**:
  - Increased risk of fibroid growth or symptom recurrence.
  - Risk of abnormal uterine bleeding.

In summary, an individualized approach, balancing the severity of menopausal symptoms with the potential risks of fibroid growth, is critical for optimal outcomes. When in doubt, consider a multidisciplinary discussion involving a gynecologist.

(L) MHT in Women with Bronchial Asthma

Managing Menopause Hormone Therapy (MHT) in women with asthma requires careful consideration of the interplay between hormonal changes and asthma control. Estrogen and progesterone levels can influence airway reactivity and inflammation, which may exacerbate or alleviate asthma symptoms depending on individual responses.

Key Considerations for MHT in Asthmatic Women:

- **Hormonal Influence on Asthma:**

- Estrogen may have a dual role in asthma, with both pro-inflammatory and anti-inflammatory effects depending on dosage and individual factors.

- Progesterone can potentially enhance respiratory muscle function but may also lead to fluid retention, potentially worsening symptoms in some cases.

- **Choice of Therapy:**
  - **Estrogen-only MHT:** Suitable for women who have undergone a hysterectomy. Transdermal estrogen is preferred, as it has a lesser impact on systemic inflammation and is less likely to exacerbate asthma symptoms.

  - **Combined Estrogen-Progesterone MHT:** For women with an intact uterus, progesterone should be carefully chosen. Micronized progesterone is generally better tolerated than synthetic progestins.

- **Mode of Delivery:**
  - **Transdermal MHT (patches, gels):** Recommended as it bypasses the liver and minimizes systemic effects, reducing the risk of worsening asthma symptoms.

  - **Oral MHT:** Should be approached with caution, as it can potentially affect asthma control more significantly.

- **Monitoring and Individualization:**
  - Women with asthma should be closely monitored for changes in symptoms after initiating MHT. Adjustments to asthma management may be necessary.

  - Regular assessment of lung function and symptom control is essential.

- **Contraindications and Risks:**
  - Severe uncontrolled asthma may require stabilization before initiating MHT.

  - Any signs of an exacerbation or adverse effects must prompt a reevaluation of the therapy.

- **Lifestyle Modifications and Adjunct Therapies:**
  - Encourage a healthy lifestyle, including smoking cessation and regular exercise, which can improve both asthma and menopausal symptoms.

  - Supplemental treatments such as inhaled corticosteroids should be optimized to manage asthma effectively.

In summary, MHT can be safely administered in women with asthma, but a personalized approach is crucial. Collaboration between gynecologists and pulmonologists ensures optimal care, balancing the benefits of MHT for menopausal symptoms with the effective management of asthma. Transdermal options and vigilant monitoring are key strategies to ensure both asthma control and menopausal relief.

(M) MHT in Women with Parkinsonism

Managing Menopause Hormone Therapy (MHT) in women with Parkinsonism requires a multidisciplinary approach due to the interplay between hormonal changes, neurodegenerative processes, and potential drug interactions.

Key Considerations for MHT in Parkinsonism:

- **Hormonal Influence on Parkinson's Disease (PD):**
    - Estrogen has neuroprotective properties, potentially influencing dopamine synthesis, release, and metabolism. However, its role in Parkinsonism remains complex and individual-specific.
    - Postmenopausal estrogen deficiency may exacerbate motor and non-motor symptoms, such as bradykinesia, rigidity, mood disturbances, and cognitive decline.
- **Benefits of MHT:**
    - **Motor Symptoms:** Limited evidence suggests that estrogen may offer modest improvement in motor function for some women with PD.
    - **Cognitive and Mood Symptoms:** Estrogen therapy might help alleviate mood disorders, such as depression and anxiety, which are common in Parkinsonism. It may also have a role in delaying cognitive decline.
- **Potential Risks and Challenges:**
    - **Thromboembolic Risk:** Women with Parkinsonism are often less mobile, increasing their risk of venous thromboembolism (VTE), which must be considered when prescribing oral MHT.
    - **Neuropsychiatric Effects:** Synthetic progestins in combined MHT can exacerbate neuropsychiatric

symptoms, such as anxiety or depression. Micronized progesterone is preferred due to its better tolerability.

   - **Drug Interactions:** Parkinson's medications, such as levodopa, may interact with MHT, potentially affecting therapeutic efficacy.

- **Choice of Therapy:**
   - **Transdermal Estrogen:** Preferred over oral routes as it minimizes first-pass metabolism and reduces thrombotic risk. It provides stable hormone levels that may benefit neurological symptoms.

   - **Progesterone:** For women with an intact uterus, micronized progesterone is recommended due to its minimal impact on mood and motor symptoms.

- **Monitoring and Individualization:**
   - Close monitoring of Parkinsonian symptoms (motor and non-motor) is necessary after initiating MHT to identify any changes in symptom severity or therapy response.

   - Regular follow-up with both a neurologist and gynecologist ensure comprehensive care and timely adjustments.

- **Non-Hormonal Alternatives:**
   - In women for whom MHT is contraindicated, non-hormonal options for managing menopausal symptoms (e.g., SSRIs, SNRIs, or gabapentin) should be considered. These may also complement PD symptom management.

- **Lifestyle and Adjunctive Measures:**
   - Encourage regular physical activity, which benefits both menopausal symptoms and Parkinson's management.

- A diet rich in antioxidants and omega-3 fatty acids may support overall neurological health.

In summary, MHT in women with Parkinsonism should be tailored to individual needs, balancing the potential neuroprotective effects of estrogen with the risks associated with therapy. Transdermal estrogen and micronized progesterone are preferred options, with close interdisciplinary collaboration to optimize outcomes for both menopausal and Parkinsonian symptoms.

(N) Should MHT Be Promoted As *"ELIXIR OF YOUTH"* In Asymptomatic Postmenopausal Women???

Menopause Hormone Therapy (MHT) in Asymptomatic Women: A Critical Perspective

The notion of using Menopause Hormone Therapy (MHT) as an **"elixir of youth"** is not supported by evidence-based medicine and should be approached with caution. While MHT offers significant benefits for managing menopausal symptoms and preventing certain age-related conditions, its use in **asymptomatic women** remains controversial and is generally **not recommended** unless specific health benefits outweigh the risks.

Evidence-Based Approach to MHT in Asymptomatic Women:

- **Primary Indication**: MHT is approved for:
  - Relief of moderate-to-severe **vasomotor symptoms** (e.g., hot flashes, night sweats).
  - Prevention and treatment of **osteoporosis** in women at high risk of fracture who cannot use other therapies.
- **No Universal Role for "Anti-Aging"**:
  - MHT does not prevent aging but addresses symptoms associated with hormonal changes during menopause.
  - Claims that MHT reverses aging or serves as a panacea for youthfulness are misleading and lack robust evidence.

Risks of MHT in Asymptomatic Women:

- **Hormone-Dependent Risks**:
  - Increased risk of **breast cancer**, particularly with combined estrogen-progesterone therapy in long-term use.
  - Potential risk of **endometrial hyperplasia** or cancer with unopposed estrogen in women with an intact uterus.
  - Increased risk of **venous thromboembolism (VTE)**, **stroke**, and, in some cases, **cardiovascular events**.
- **Unnecessary Exposure**:
  - In asymptomatic women, the risks of MHT may outweigh benefits since the therapy does not address any pressing clinical need.

Addressing the "Elixir of Youth" Misconception:

- **Marketing vs. Reality**:
  - Some promotional agencies exaggerate MHT's benefits for anti-aging to attract consumers.
  - This portrayal undermines the evidence-based framework for MHT and risks exposing women to unnecessary health hazards.
- **Ethical Considerations**:
  - Physicians and healthcare providers have a responsibility to educate women about the realistic benefits and risks of MHT.
  - Decisions about MHT should be guided by clinical need, not societal pressures or marketing strategies.

Alternatives to MHT for "Youthful Aging"

- For asymptomatic women concerned about aging, non-hormonal approaches should be emphasized:
  - **Lifestyle Modifications**:
    Regular exercise, a balanced diet, adequate sleep, and stress management.

  - **Nutritional Support**:
    Adequate calcium, vitamin D, and omega-3 fatty acids.

  - **Cosmetic Interventions**:
    Topical treatments (e.g., retinoids) or aesthetic procedures for skin health, which are safer and targeted.

Patient-Centered Decision-Making

- Women considering MHT should receive balanced, evidence-based information about its benefits and risks.

- Decisions should focus on **quality of life, individual risk factors**, and preferences rather than societal pressures or marketing claims.

In summary, MHT should not be used routinely in asymptomatic women as a preventive or anti-aging treatment. The portrayal of MHT as an "elixir of youth" is both scientifically unfounded and ethically problematic. Healthcare providers must advocate for evidence-based use, educate women about realistic expectations, and ensure that decisions about MHT are driven by medical need, not marketing hype.

CHAPTER VIII: FUTURE DIRECTIONS

"Progress is impossible without change,

and those who cannot change their minds

cannot change anything."

– George Bernard Shaw

(A) Historical Challenges with MHT

- **Past Controversies:**
  - Misinterpretation of studies like the Women's Health Initiative (WHI), leading to fear of risks (e.g., breast cancer, cardiovascular disease).
  - Lack of differentiation between risks of combined vs. estrogen-only therapy.
- **Irrational Use:**
  - Overprescription without proper patient stratification in the past.
  - Inappropriate dosing and regimens without evidence-based protocols.

(A) Current Barriers to MHT Use

- **Gynecologists' Hesitation**
  - Lack of updated knowledge on MHT indications and safety.
  - Preference for money-yielding fields like laparoscopic surgery and infertility treatment.

- **Integration into Primary Care:**
  Train primary care physicians to initiate and monitor MHT.

- **Collaboration with Professional Bodies**
  - Strengthen partnerships with organizations like:
    - International Menopause Society (IMS).
    - North American Menopause Society (NAMS).
    - National Obstetrics and Gynecology Societies.

- **Addressing Ethical and Economic Aspects**
  - **Ethical Practice:**
    Emphasize the importance of patient-centered care over revenue-driven practices.

  - **Cost-Effective Solutions:**
    Promote affordable formulations and public health subsidies for MHT.

- **Cultural and Regional Adaptation**
  - **Tailored Messaging:**
    Address cultural stigmas around menopause in developing countries.

  - **Local Language Resources:**
    Develop education material in regional languages.

- **Long-Term Vision**
  - **Normalization of Menopause Management:**
    Integrate menopause care as a routine part of women's health.

  - **Global Advocacy:**
    WHO and similar organizations to endorse and promote menopausal health as a public health priority.

CHAPTER IX: CONCLUSION

"Life is a journey, and every phase brings its own rewards and lessons."

– Anonymous

- **A Renewed Perspective on MHT:**

  Menopause Hormone Therapy has undergone significant evolution in its understanding, application, and outcomes. Today, MHT is no longer viewed through the lens of past controversies but as a precise, evidence-based treatment tailored to individual patient needs. Modern research has clarified its benefits and risks, enabling informed decisions that prioritize patient safety and quality of life.

- **Benefits of MHT in Specific Contexts:**

  - **Symptom Management:** MHT remains the gold standard for alleviating vasomotor symptoms (hot flashes, night sweats), genitourinary syndrome, and improving sleep and mood in menopausal women.

  - **Bone Health:** It plays a pivotal role in preventing osteoporosis and reducing fracture risk in postmenopausal women at high risk of bone density loss.

  - **Cardiovascular and Metabolic Health:** Recent evidence suggests that initiating MHT early in menopause (within the "timing hypothesis window") for vasomotor symptoms may have favorable effects on cardiovascular health and metabolic parameters.

- **Individualized Therapy for Optimal Outcomes:**

  Modern MHT emphasizes a personalized approach, considering factors such as age, menopausal stage, symptom severity, comorbid conditions (e.g., diabetes, hypertension), and patient preferences. This ensures that therapy is both effective and safe.

- **Risk calculations are applied strictly:**

  - Taking detailed history.
  - Physical examination, including breast and pelvis.
  - Basic mandatory investigations.
  - Special added investigations for some women, if indicated as per history.
  - Using “Risk Assessment Tools” for breast cancer and cardiovascular disease.
  - Using the right MHT, route, and duration of therapy.

- **Addressing Misconceptions and Reassuring Practitioners:**

  - **The controversies** surrounding MHT, largely stemming from its irrelevant or non-individualized use in the past, have been clarified through extensive research. Current guidelines and clinical practices are based on robust data, dispelling myths and reinforcing confidence among medical practitioners in prescribing MHT.
  - **Encouraging Patient-Physician Collaboration** Open communication between patients and physicians is critical. Educating women about

menopause, MHT options, and their associated benefits and risks fosters trust and allows for shared decision-making, ensuring that therapy aligns with the patient's health goals.

- **Future Directions in MHT:**

  Continued research, especially in understanding long-term effects and tailoring therapies further (e.g., non-oral routes, bioidentical hormones), will refine MHT practices. The focus remains on maximizing benefits while minimizing risks for menopausal women.

- **In Summary:**

  Menopause Hormone Therapy, when used judiciously and based on current evidence, is a safe and highly effective intervention for improving the health and well-being of menopausal women. By shifting our perspective from the controversies of the past to the advancements of today, we can confidently integrate MHT into modern medical practice. This approach ensures that women experience a fulfilling and healthy transition through menopause, supported by therapies that enhance their quality of life and mitigate long-term health risks.

"Right Woman, Right MHT, Right Dose,

and Right Duration

is the Right Approach for Prescribing MHT

so that Benefits far Outweigh the Risk."

For asymptomatic women, aging healthfully and gracefully is best achieved through lifestyle changes, preventive healthcare, and addressing specific health concerns individually and not by assuming MHT as "Elixir of Youth".

CHAPTER X: REFERENCES

1. Clinical Practice on menopause – Indian Menopause Society.

2. Journal of Mid Life Health.

3. Menopause and MHT in 2024: addressing the key controversies – an International Menopause Society White Paper. (https://doi.org/10.1080/13697137.2024.2394950)

4. Dinnerstein L, Dudley EC, Hopper JL et. al. A prospective population-based study of menopause symptoms. Obstet. Gynecol 2000; 96:351.

5.Woods NF, Mitchell ES. Symptoms during the menopause: prevalence, severity and significance in women's lives. Am J Med 2005; 118 suppl 12 B: 14.

6. National Institute of Health State-of-the-Science Conference Statement: management of menopause-related symptoms. Ann Intern Med 2005; 142:1003.

7. Kronenberg F. Hot flashes: epidemiology and physiology. Ann N Y Acad Sci 1090; 592:52.

8. McKinley SM. The normal menopause transition: an overview. Maturitas 1996; 23:137.

9. Cohen LS, Soars CN, Joffe H. Diagnosis and management of mood disorders during menopause transition. Am J Med 2005; 118 suppl 12B:93.

10. Freedom RR, Roehrs TA. Sleep disturbances in menopause. Menopause 2007; 14:826.

11. Mathews KA, Wings RR, Kuller LH, et.al. Influence of the perimenopause on cardiovascular risk factors and symptoms middle-aged healthy women. Arch Intern Med 1994; 154:2349.

12. Thurston RC, Joffe H. Vasomotor symptoms and menopause: findings from the study of women's health across the nation. Obstet. Gynecol Clin North Am 2011; 38:489.

13. Mohyi D, Tabassi K, Simon J. Differential diagnosis of hot flashes. Maturitas 1997; 27:203.

14. Anklesaria BS. Why should it be the stage of menopause? Modern management of menopause with isoflavones; 2007.PP. 7-9.

15. Anklesaria BS. Staging of Menopause. The Menopause FOGSI Focus; 2010. PP. 3 – 5.

16. Harlow SD, Gass M, Hall JE, et.al. Executive summary of the stages of reproductive aging workshop + 10: addressing the unfinished agenda of staging reproductive aging. Fertil Steril. 2012;97(4):843-51.

17. Brown WJ, Mishra GD, Dobson A. Changes in physical symptoms during the menopause transition. Int J Behav Med 2002;9(1):53-67.

18. Barton DL, Loprinzi C, Atherton PJ, et. al. Dehydroepiandrosterone for the treatment of hot flashes: A pilot study. Support cancer then 2006;3(2):91-7.

19. Calleja-Agius J, Brincat M. Urogenital atrophy. Climacteric 2009; 12:279-285.

20. MacBride M, Rhodes D, Shuster L. Vulvovaginal atrophy. Mayo Clin Proc 2010; 85:87-94.

21. Portman D, Gass M, Vulvovaginal Atrophy Terminology Consensus Conference Panel. Genitourinary Syndrome of Menopause: new terminology of vulvovaginal atrophy from International Society for the Study of Women's Sexual Health and the North American Menopause Society. Menopause 2014;21(10);1063-1068.

22. Palacios S. Managing urogenital atrophy. Maturitas 2009;63(4):315-318.

23. Lester J, Pahouja G, Aderson B, Lustberg M. Atrophic vaginitis in breast cancer survivors: a difficult survivorship issue. J Pers Med 2015;5(2):50-66.

24. NICE. Menopause: diagnosis and management of genitourinary syndrome of menopause. NICE Guidelines 23. NICE, 2015. Available at: www.nice.org.uk/ng23.

25. Therapies for the management of genitourinary syndrome of menopause. Palacios S, Combalia J, Emsellem C, Gaslain Y, Khorsandi D. Post Repro Health. 2020;26:32-42. (PubMed) (Google Scholar).

26. ACOG Practice Bulletin No. 141: management of menopausal symptoms. American College of Obstetrician and Gynaecologist. Obstet Gynecol. 2014;123:202-216, (PubMed) (Google Scholar).

27. Genitourinary changes with aging. Mitchell CM, Waetjen LE. Obstet Gynecol Clin North Am. 2018;45:737-750. (PubMed) (Google Scholar).

28. The role of local vaginal oestrogen for treatment of vaginal atrophy in postmenopausal women:2007 position statement of the North American Society. Menopause 2007;14:355-369. (PubMed) (Google Scholar).

29. Genitourinary Syndrome of Menopause: common problem, effective treatments. Phillips NA, Bachmann GA. Cleve Clin J Med. 2018;85:390-398. (PubMed) (Google Scholar).

30. Genitourinary Syndrome of menopause. Briggs P. Post Report Health. 2019:2053369119884144. (PubMed) (Google Scholar).

31. Genitourinary syndrome of menopause: an overview of clinical manifestations, pathophysiology, aetiology, evaluation and management. Gandhi J, Chen A, Dagur G, Suh Y, Smit N, Cali B, Khan SA, Am J Obstet Gynecol. 2016;215:504-711. (PubMed) (Google Scholar).

32. Yasuda H. RANKL, a necessary chance for clinical application to osteoporosis and cancer-related bone disease. World J Orthop. 2013;4:207-217.(PMC free article) (PubMed) (Google Scholar).

33. Sambrook P, Cooper C. Osteoporosis. Lancet. 2006;368:2010-2018 (Pub Med) (Google Scholar).

34. Rossini M, Adami S, Bertoldo F, et.al. Guidelines for the diagnosis, prevention and management of osteoporosis. Reumatismo. 2016;68:1-39. (PubMed) (Google Scholar).

35. Bauer JS, Link TM. Advances in osteoporosis imaging. Europ J Radiol. 2009;71:440-449 (PubMed) (Google Scholar).

36. National Osteoporosis Foundation, 2013 Clinician's Guide for prevention and treatment. http://nof/public/contenr/resource/913/files/580.pdf (Accepted on November 14, 2013).

37. American Association of Clinical Endocrinologists Medical Guidelines for clinical practice for the diagnosis and treatment of postmenopausal osteoporosis.

38. Global AL, Laya MB (May 2015), "Osteoporosis: screening, prevention and management." The Medical Clinics of North America. 99(3):587-606. Doi:10. 1016/j.mcna. 2015.01.010. PMID 25841602.

39. Clinical Challenges: Managing osteoporosis in male hypogonadism. www.medpagetoday.com. 4 June 2018. Retrieved 22 March 2022.

40. Rigo J, et.al Reference values of body composition obtained by dual x-ray absorptiometry in preterm and term neonates. J Pediatr Gastroenterol Nutr. 1998;27:184-90. (PubMed) (Google Scholar).

41. Hlaing TT, Compston JE. Biochemical markers of bone turnover-uses and limitations. Ann Clin Biochem 2014; 51:189.

42. Bauer D, Krege J, Lane N, et.al. National Bone Health Alliance Bone Turnover Marker Project: current practices and the need for US harmonization, standardization and common reference ranges. Osteoporosis Int 2o12;23:2425.

43. The NAMS 2017 Hormone Therapy Position Statement Advisory Panel. The 2017 hormone therapy position statement of the North American Menopause Society. Menopause 2017;24:728.

44. Steingold KA, Laufer L, Chetkowski RJ, et.al. Treatment of hot flashes with transdermal estradiol administration. J Clin Endocrinol Metab 1985;61:627.

45. Nelson HD. Commonly used types of postmenopausal oestrogen for treatment of hot flashes: scientific review. JAWA 2004; 291:1610.

46. North American Menopause Society. The 2012 hormone position statement of: The North American Menopause Society. Menopause 2012;19:257.

47. Sood R, Faubion SS, Kuhle CL et.al prescribing Menopause Therapy: an evidence-based approach. Int. J Women's Health 2014;6:47.

48. Udoff L, Langenberg P, Adashi EY. Combined Continuous Hormone Replacement Therapy: a critical review. Obstet Gynecol 1995;86:306.

49. ACOG Practice Bulletin No. 141: management of menopausal symptoms. Obstet Gynecol. 2014;123(1):202-216.

50. Bakour SH, Williamson J. Latest evidence on using hormone therapy in the menopause. Obstet Gynecol, 2014.

51. The 2022 hormone therapy position statement of the North American Menopause Society. Menopause (New York). 2022;29(7):767-794.

Previous Books Published in the Series, "Women's Health"

All books are available on Amazon.in as well as on Amazon.com.

Universal Link:

https://relinks.me/BoBW6ZVMXY

1. **Preconception Care Makes a Difference**

"Preconception Care and Counselling is the window of opportunity to tackle all unhealthy maternal problems resulting in favorable environment for the growth of embryo/fetus."

"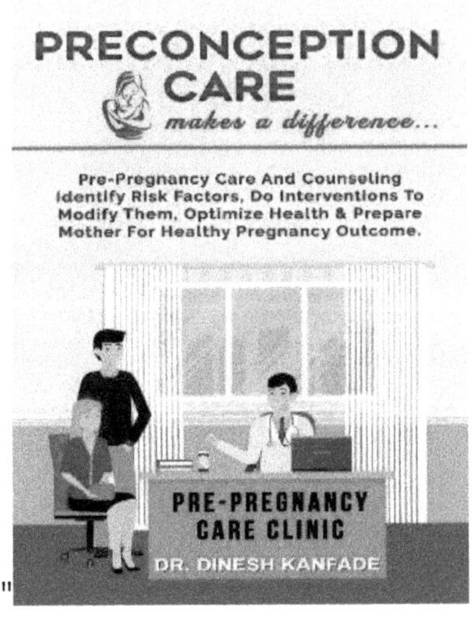

2. **Understanding Menopause**

"The biggest achievement of the last century is greater longevity that has resulted in an increased aged population worldwide. But the advantage of increased longevity is only when it is translated into healthy aging. Discover the secrets for understanding and managing menopause, thereby improving quality of life with this comprehensive updated guide."

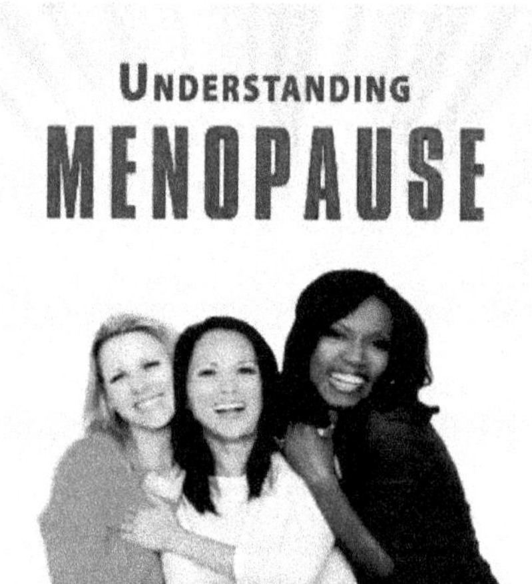

3. **Heart and Bone Health**

"We are living in aged population worldwide. It is obvious that women live significant part of their life after menopause. The ovaries of long years of dedicated service, have not the ability of retiring gracefully. But because of estrogen deficiency, ovaries become irritable and transmits this irritation to various organs of the body resulting in non-communicable diseases such as cardiovascular disease and osteoporosis. The advantage of increased longevity is only when it is translated into healthy aging. With a healthy lifestyle and understanding the pathophysiology of cardiovascular disease and osteoporosis in postmenopausal women, not only years will be added to increase the lifespan, but the extra years added will be of good quality. Discover the secretes of managing heart and bone health in postmenopausal women, thereby improving quality of life with this comprehensive guide."

POSTMENOPAUSAL

HEART & BONE HEALTH

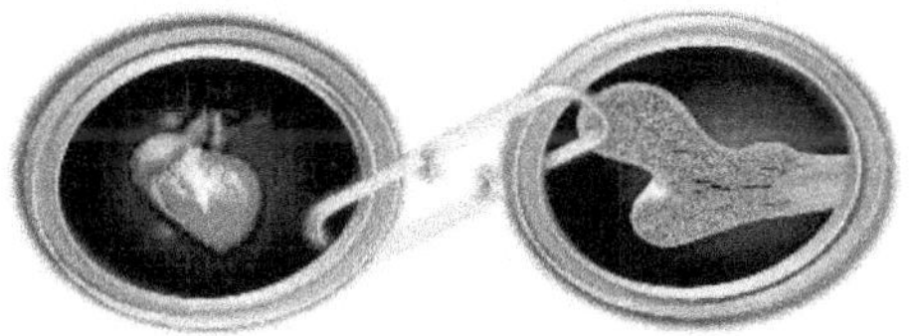

Empowering Women To Take Charge Of Their Health By Adopting Healthy Lifestyles For A Vibrant Life Beyond Menopause

DR. DINESH KANFADE

4. **Embracing Postmenopausal Intimacy**

"The postmenopausal phase, with its unique challenges and opportunities stands as a testament to the resilience of human intimacy. It is within this period of transformation that find an invitation to redefine and to rediscover physical closeness. Don't miss out on the transformative wisdom within these pages. Embrace the journey towards vibrant and fulfilling postmenopausal intimacy."

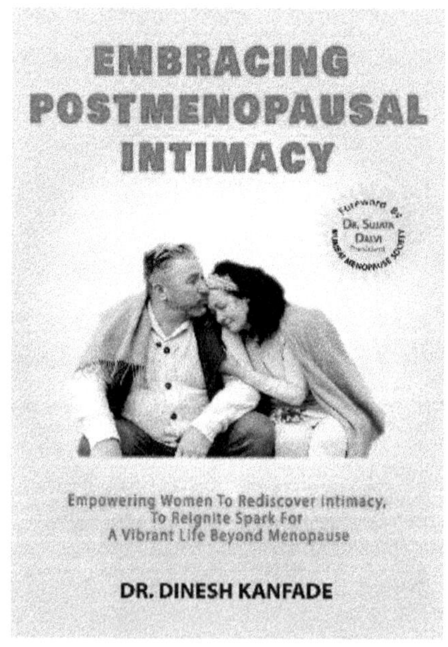

5. **Menstrual Health and Hygiene**

Unlock the secrets to optimal menstrual health and hygiene in this comprehensive guide.
From debunking myths to empowering insights, this book offers practical tips and evidence-based strategies for every stage of menstruation.

Whether you are seeking solutions for menstrual discomfort, navigating hygiene products or simply aiming for a healthier menstrual cycle, this book has covered everything you want in relation to menstruation.

Together, let us embark on this journey of enlightment, guided by the wisdom contained within these pages.

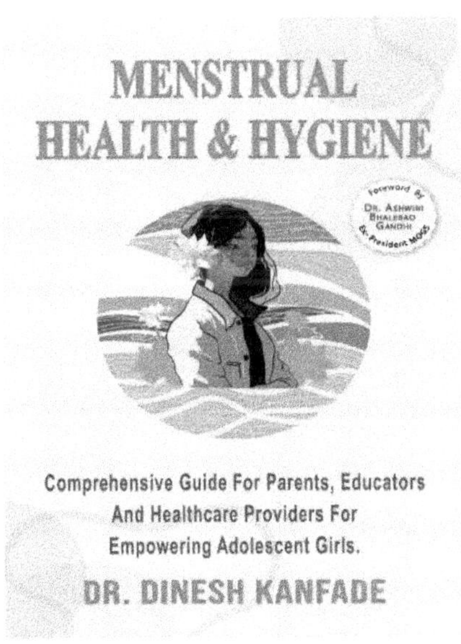

6. **The Silent Struggles: Understanding Women's Mental Health**

Mental health is often a quiet battle, and for women, it is a journey through the unique challenges at every stage of life.

The book is a comprehensive exploration of the emotional and psychological hurdles women face- from adolescence, through their reproductive years, to menopause.

The recurrence of heinous acts such as recent physical and sexual assault of junior doctor R. G. Kar Medical College Kolkata (August 2024), the infamous Nirbhaya case (2012) and many others suggest several concerning ground realities.

This book offers a profound understanding of how social, cultural and biological factors shape a woman's mental health.

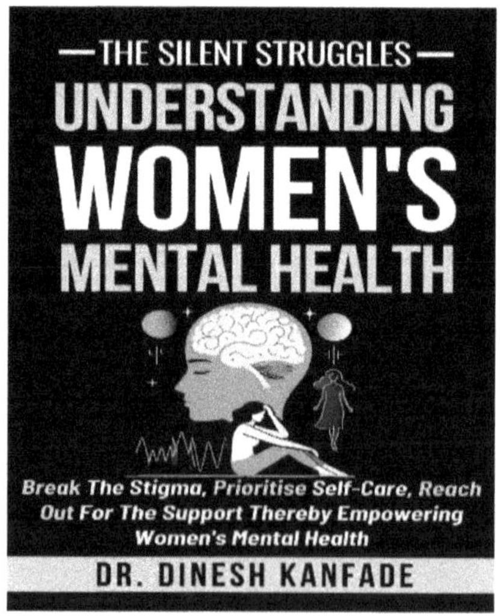

7. **Nurturing Wellness: The Path to Breast Cancer Awareness**

The breast has always been the symbol of womanhood and ultimate fertility. As a result, both disease and surgery of the breast evoke a fear of mutilation and loss of femininity.

Breast cancer remains a major health concern due to its high incidence worldwide and the significant impact it has on women's health.

This book contains vital information about the prevalence, prevention and tips for early detection of breast cancer for better survival rates.

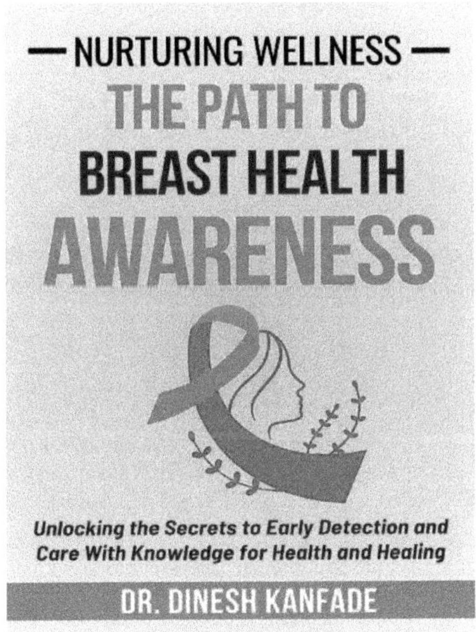

8. **Nurturing Wellness: The Path to Postmenopausal Heart Disease Awareness**

The biggest achievement of the last century is greater longevity that has resulted in increasing aged population worldwide. It is obvious that women have to live significant part of their lives after menopause. Menopause transition bring profound hormonal changes that can affect multiple aspects of health, including an often-overlooked issue: cardiovascular disease (CVD). Heart disease is the leading cause of death among women in postmenopausal age group, cancer being second. Yet many women are unaware of the heightened risk of CVD they face after menopause. The benefit of increased lifespan is only when it is translated into healthy aging.

— NURTURING WELLNESS —
THE PATH TO
POSTMENOPAUSAL
HEART DISEASE AWARENESS

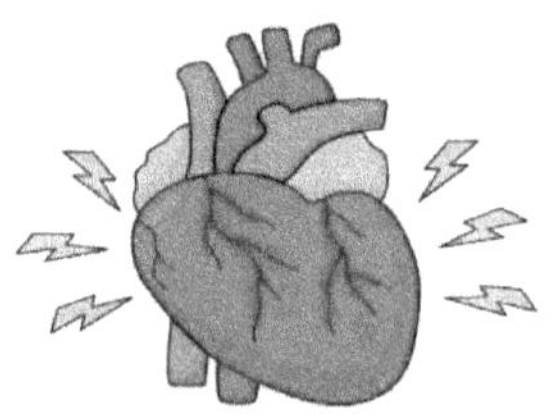

Empowering Women to Understand Menopause and Heart Health, Taking Control for a Vibrant Life Beyond Menopause

DR. DINESH KANFADE

9. Nurturing Wellness: The Path to Postmenopausal Osteoporosis Awareness

Osteoporosis is frequently called the "Silent Killer" because it itself has no symptoms. The patients are unaware of their bone loss until they experience a fracture.

With aging, bone density naturally decreases in both genders, but for many women, this process accelerates after menopause due to estrogen deficiency, leading to brittle bones, subsequent fractures, and a significant impact on quality of life. Despite its widespread prevalence, osteoporosis remains an often-overlooked health issue, overshadowed by other conditions.

The rapid bone loss typically starts within the first 5 - 7 years after menopause, with women losing up to 20% of their bone mass during this period.

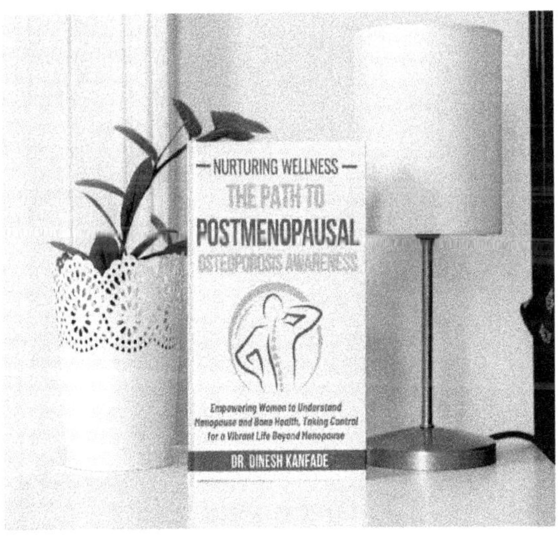

www.ingramcontent.com/pod-product-compliance
Lightning Source LLC
LaVergne TN
LVHW021137160826
845679LV00023B/1940